"The book is gentle and reassuring—the authors provide encouragement at every step. At first I was nervous about doing the exercises, but after an hour I could barely write fast enough! One very valuable part of this book is how it helps you distinguish between facts, thoughts, and feelings, and exactly how to deal with each of them. Highly recommended."
—**Linda H., Saskatoon, Canada**

"This is the PTSD self-help book I've been waiting for. Not everyone is able to see a therapist. The strategies in this book are informed by extensive research and are written in a way that makes them easy to understand and use." —**Debra Kaysen, PhD, ABPP, Department of Psychiatry and Behavioral Sciences, Stanford University**

"If you want to take back your life from PTSD, this book is a gift. The authors are psychologists with many years of clinical experience among them, who write with warmth and compassion." —**Tara E. Galovski, PhD, Director, Women's Health Sciences Division, National Center for PTSD; Department of Psychiatry, Boston University Chobanian and Avedisian School of Medicine**

"I love this workbook—it's super solid. Besides the information being sound and smart, the way it is presented is perfect. The worksheets and exercises helped make complex, overwhelming emotional issues feel more approachable, so I could understand and work through them." —**Mary C., Chicago**

"Cognitive processing therapy (CPT) is a truly groundbreaking treatment. This practical, informed, and compassionate workbook teaches you to identify and change the stuck points that trap you in the past, so you can cope better and overcome guilt, fear, and helplessness. This is a book that every trauma survivor should have. It not only will make lives better, but in some cases will save lives." —**Robert L. Leahy, PhD, author of** *If Only . . .*

"Decades of research have shown that CPT is a highly effective treatment. This easy-to-read self-help guide puts the tools for recovery directly into your hands. It is filled with relatable scenarios, tried-and-tested techniques, and helpful solutions." —**Reginald D. V. Nixon, PhD, College of Education, Psychology, and Social Work, and Flinders University Institute for Mental Health and Wellbeing, Flinders University, Australia**

"CPT enables trauma survivors not only to recover from PTSD, but also to enjoy increased resilience in the face of future stressors and life challenges. Now the developer of CPT, together with her master clinician colleagues, shares this remarkable approach to PTSD recovery directly with readers who may lack access to a formally trained CPT therapist. Invaluable!" —**Ann M. Rasmusson, MD, Department of Psychiatry, Boston University Chobanian and Avedisian School of Medicine**

Getting Unstuck from PTSD

Also Available

FOR PROFESSIONALS

Cognitive Processing Therapy for PTSD:
A Comprehensive Manual
Patricia A. Resick, Candice M. Monson, Kathleen M. Chard

Getting Unstuck from PTSD

USING COGNITIVE PROCESSING THERAPY TO GUIDE YOUR RECOVERY

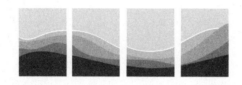

Patricia A. Resick, PhD

Shannon Wiltsey Stirman, PhD

Stefanie T. LoSavio, PhD

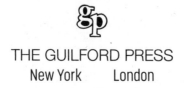

THE GUILFORD PRESS

New York   London

Printed in the United States of America

Last digit is print number: 9   8   7   6   5   4   3

Library of Congress Cataloging-in-Publication Data

Names: Resick, Patricia A., author. | Wiltsey Stirman, Shannon, author. |
  LoSavio, Stefanie T., author.
Title: Getting unstuck from PTSD : using cognitive processing therapy to guide
  your recovery / Patricia A. Resick, PhD, Shannon Wiltsey Stirman, PhD,
  Stefanie T. LoSavio, PhD.
Description: New York : The Guilford Press, [2023] | Includes bibliographical references
  and index.
Identifiers: LCCN 2023009544 | ISBN 9781462551460 (hardcover) | ISBN
  9781462549832 (paperback)
Subjects: LCSH: Post-traumatic stress disorder—Treatment—Popular works. | Cognitive
  therapy—Popular works. | BISAC: PSYCHOLOGY / Psychopathology /
  Post-Traumatic Stress Disorder (PTSD) | RELIGION / Counseling
Classification: LCC RC552.P67 R4684 2023 | DDC 616.85/21—dc23/eng/20230414
LC record available at *https://lccn.loc.gov/2023009544*

To three of the finest men I know,
Keith, Marty, and Matt Shaw

—P. A. R.

To my children, Henry, Eve, and Brahm,
and to the friends and family whose love and support
have helped me through the toughest times

—S. W. S.

To my family,
especially John, Susan, Candy, and Chris LoSavio;
Renis Pavlik; and David and William Schreiber;
and in memory of Lawrence Cohen and Patricia Schreiber

—S. T. L.

Contents

Authors' Note

Illustrations are composites of real individuals or otherwise thoroughly disguised to protect privacy.

Some of the content of this workbook is based on the following sources:

P. A. Resick, C. M. Monson, and K. M. Chard (2017). *Cognitive Processing Therapy for PTSD: A Comprehensive Manual.* New York: Guilford Press. Copyright © 2017 The Guilford Press. Used by permission.

S. T. LoSavio (2017). Cognitive Processing Therapy—Modular Version (CPT-M). In *Therapist Manual and Client Materials.* Unpublished manuscript, Duke University Medical Center, Durham, NC. Copyright © 2017 Stefanie T. LoSavio. Used by permission.

P. A. Resick, S. Wiltsey Stirman, and K. Dondanville (2021). *Messaging-Based Cognitive Processing Therapy Manual and Client Materials.* Unpublished manuscript. Copyright © 2021. Used by permission.

Acknowledgments

First, we would like to thank all of the courageous trauma survivors who we have worked with for sharing your stories and letting us accompany you on your journey toward healing.

This book would not be possible without the all-star power of Candice M. Monson, PhD, and Kathleen M. Chard, PhD, who coauthored with Patricia Resick the cognitive processing therapy (CPT) manual for therapists in its various iterations, starting with the early U.S. Department of Veterans Affairs manual of 2007 through the comprehensive manual whose second edition is now underway with The Guilford Press. Their open-mindedness to feedback and continual striving to make the therapist manual more accessible to providers and clients were an inspiration to us as we crafted this book for people suffering from posttraumatic stress disorder (PTSD).

We hope that as people work the program in these pages they will feel the collective efforts of many people from the past 35 years, since the inception of CPT for PTSD. The number of other researchers, trainers, therapists, coordinators, and supervisors who have contributed in one way or another to the effectiveness and spread of CPT in the United States and throughout the world is too great to name here. Let us just say, the "it takes a village" expression is a great understatement.

Our editors at Guilford, Kitty Moore, Chris Benton, and Anna Brackett, provided valuable insights and suggestions at every step of the way. We appreciate their efforts and those of the many others at Guilford who have worked behind the scenes to help this book take shape.

Finally, we want to express our deep gratitude to our families and friends. The support you have shown for our work over the years means the world to us.

Getting Unstuck from PTSD

Part I

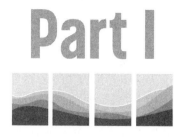

Introduction

How People Get Stuck in PTSD and How to Get Unstuck

Welcome! If you have experienced traumatic events in your life, you are not alone. Most people experience one or more traumatic events at some point, like physical or sexual abuse, combat, an accident, or the traumatic and unexpected loss of a loved one. For some, however, the traumatic experience lingers with them for a long time afterward, and they get "stuck" in their recovery from the event, experiencing symptoms of posttraumatic stress disorder (PTSD).

Margaret was physically abused by her ex-husband and has struggled with self-blame, thinking "It's my fault because I stayed," and difficulty trusting others since the trauma. She has often felt lonely and wished she could have a fulfilling romantic relationship but has struggled to let anyone get close to her again out of fear that she will be abused again.

Joseph's brother died by a drug overdose, and, ever since, he has struggled with guilt about living his life when his brother is not around to live his. He also often ruminates about how he might have prevented his brother's death if he had been with him. This experience has made it difficult for Joseph to focus on his life today and enjoy time with his children.

Cynthia was sexually abused as a child and also experienced sexual assault later on as an adolescent and as an adult. Because she was repeatedly taken advantage of in this way, she has sometimes wondered if her only value is to meet other people's needs, and she has struggled to set boundaries with others out of

1

concern that they will leave her if she doesn't comply with their wishes. This has caused problems for her both in her personal relationships and at work.

These examples demonstrate the impact trauma can have on a person's life and how it can continue to cause problems even years later. Some questions to consider are:

- Have you had trouble getting back to yourself after a life-threatening or violating experience? Has it interfered with work or relationships?
- Have you gotten stuck second-guessing what you did or did not do or trying to think of ways the event might have been prevented?
- Have you found yourself trying hard not to think about what happened or avoiding reminders of the event?

If you have had problems like these, you may be dealing with symptoms of PTSD. The good news is that recovery is possible. This book is designed to help people who have gotten stuck with symptoms of PTSD get unstuck and back to living their lives today.

In the chapters that follow, you'll be introduced to this book, which is a comprehensive approach to help you get unstuck from PTSD. You'll also learn more about why people get stuck in PTSD and how to get unstuck using the strategies in this book. Finally, you'll have an opportunity to make a plan to process your trauma so that you can get back to living your life focused on the things that matter to you.

1

Overview of This Book

We're so glad you have found your way to this book and that you are interested in addressing your trauma.

This book is for you if you . . .

- ✓ Have experienced one or more traumatic events.
- ✓ Have been bothered by symptoms of PTSD, such as unwanted thoughts or memories of your trauma(s), strong emotional or physical reactions to reminders, or wanting to avoid thinking about the trauma memory.
- ✓ Are willing to face your traumatic experience(s) so you can move toward recovery.
- ✓ Are willing to make it a priority to spend time practicing the skills you learn.

This book will walk you through a comprehensive approach to overcome your trauma and get back to living the life you want to lead. It's not necessary to have a formal diagnosis of PTSD to use this book. In the next chapter, you'll complete a questionnaire to self-assess your PTSD symptoms.

This book contains all the worksheets and tools you'll need to recover from your traumatic experiences. By working on the trauma a little each day, you can make progress toward taking back your life. Some people complete this program in a few weeks, and some take up to several months. It all depends on your own pacing. When people undergo trauma-focused treatments with therapists, though, research has shown that working consistently over a shorter period of time (two to three months) can lead to better results than spreading it out over a longer period of time.

Working on your trauma won't make the memory go away, but it will reduce its hold on you so you can begin to move forward. Instead of being blindsided by the trauma memory when you least expect it, you might be able to think about it when you want to without all the strong negative emotions and the sense that the traumatic event is happening all over again. That means that you can get back to living your life in the here-and-now, without your trauma(s) impairing your relationships or your ability to achieve your goals.

～～～ What Is Cognitive Processing Therapy? ～～～

This book is based on cognitive processing therapy (CPT), which is one of the most effective therapies for PTSD. CPT is an approach that helps people get unstuck from their PTSD and move toward recovery. The goals of CPT are to improve your PTSD and related symptoms, such as depression, anxiety, guilt, and shame. It also aims to improve your day-to-day functioning. CPT helps you figure out where you got stuck in your recovery from the trauma (such as unfairly blaming yourself for what happened or not preventing it) and helps you get unstuck by examining the facts of the trauma so that you can make sense of your experience and recover.

CPT is effective. Many research studies have demonstrated that CPT works for people who have experienced a variety of different forms of trauma. These studies have taken place in community treatment settings, military and veteran hospitals, and in many countries. Most people who have completed CPT have had noticeable reductions in symptoms of PTSD, as well as other problems, such as depression, suicidal thoughts, hopelessness, anger, guilt, and substance use. (See the box below for details.)

Evidence for CPT

Over the decades that CPT has been developed and refined, numerous researchers and therapists have collected data to make sure it works. It has been studied in rigorous clinical trials, where it has been compared to other effective treatments, with steps in place to make sure that the effect of treatment was real and due to the treatment itself, and that the results wouldn't be biased. The first large study of CPT compared CPT to prolonged exposure, another trauma-focused treatment that had been shown to be very effective for PTSD. One hundred seventy-one women who had been raped (and most had experienced other traumas as well) began CPT or prolonged exposure. The women did equally well in both treatments, except that the women who participated in CPT reported experiencing less guilt after treatment and lower suicidal ideation. A long-term follow-up five to ten years after the posttreatment assessment found that the improvements were maintained over long periods of time. Later studies showed that some different variations of CPT (like group treatment, treatment that didn't include a written account of the trauma, and versions for people who couldn't read or write) were also very effective. Since the early studies that showed that CPT was effective, there have been almost forty carefully controlled studies comparing CPT to other therapies and continuing to show that CPT reduces PTSD and other issues like depression, suicidal thoughts, and anger. There have also been many studies that have examined predictors of treatment outcome and tests of the treatment in various therapy settings, with people who experienced different types of trauma, and in other countries and cultures. If you want to read publications of studies about CPT, a number of them are located on the CPT website (*http://cptforptsd.com*) under "Resources."

CPT works even for people who have a complex trauma history and symptoms beyond PTSD. For example, many people with PTSD also have depression or substance use issues. Research has shown that even people with additional problems like these benefit from CPT. CPT was originally developed to help rape survivors in the late 1980s, but it was quickly tested with people who have experienced a range of traumatic events, including incarcerated adolescents, women who had been sexually abused in childhood, refugees, military veterans, and many others. Most often people have more than one traumatic event in their life, and the research on CPT over the past thirty-plus years has shown that CPT works for people even if they have complex trauma histories and a complex set of symptoms. In other words, CPT was developed and tested with all types of people, and very possibly with people who struggle with some of the same issues that you struggle with.

CPT is a **time-limited, recovery-focused** approach, which means that it's not intended to go on for years and years. Instead, positive changes can often be seen in just a few weeks. This may be hard to believe if you've been suffering from PTSD for a long time, but if you stick with it and engage fully with the activities, working at it a little each day, you'll have the opportunity to see for yourself how it works.

CPT is **trauma focused.** That means that most of the time the focus is on your traumatic experiences and their impact on you. This is because trauma-focused treatments are the most effective treatments available for people with PTSD. Whereas you may have something stressful going on in your life that is at the top of your mind, focusing on day-to-day events won't treat your underlying PTSD. On the other hand, if you address your PTSD by working on the trauma, you're likely to see improvements in your day-to-day functioning. You'll also see that many of the skills and tools you learn in CPT can help you with everyday issues as well.

Why We Wrote This Book

We are psychologists with many years of experience working with people who have endured traumatic events and who suffer from PTSD. Patricia Resick originally developed CPT over thirty years ago and has trained thousands of therapists, including Shannon Wiltsey Stirman and Stefanie LoSavio, to use CPT with our clients. Now we all train students and therapists to use CPT in their clinical practice, and we have consulted on thousands of cases. However, there are still places where it is very difficult, if not impossible, to find a therapist who has been trained in CPT. We also recognize that factors like costs/lack of insurance and difficulty getting time away from work, school, or caregiving responsibilities make it hard to get to therapy on a regular basis. Other people may worry that their friends, families, or employers may not be supportive of their receiving therapy, and they feel a need to keep their PTSD to themselves. We believe that everyone should have access to tools that can help them. We wrote this book so that people who can't do CPT with a trained therapist can still have the opportunity to use CPT tools to support their recovery. It's courageous to decide to work on your PTSD, and we sincerely hope that you'll find this book helpful.

CPT has been tested and shown to be effective when delivered with a therapist in person or over the computer (such as via Zoom), and we even have evidence that it can work through a texting format. It has not been formally tested as of yet as a self-help book. However, studies have shown that self-help for PTSD can be beneficial, and we have included the same skills and organized this book as you might complete it with a therapist. We have also included a lot of extra guidance so that you can complete the exercises on your own. It is our hope that people will be able to use this book to get benefits similar to those from doing CPT with a therapist.

That said, if you get stuck, help is available. If, while using this book, you decide you could benefit from the assistance of a therapist, there are thousands of therapists who have been trained in CPT through the U.S. Department of Veterans Affairs (VA) or in the community. If you are a U.S. veteran, you can contact your local VA or Vet Center to see if you qualify for services and can ask for a CPT-trained therapist. If you are looking for someone in the community and have access to the Internet, you can go online to *http://cptforptsd.com* and click on "CPT Provider Roster." You can search by country, state, city, or zip code. If engaging in therapy by computer (Zoom or some other format), you can search for anyone who is licensed in your state. If you want to see them in person, you will need to search for someone nearby. Don't give up if the person you contact is fully booked or charges more than you can afford. That person may have a suggestion for you, and some providers or agencies have sliding fee scales or take insurance or Medicaid.

Getting Unstuck

Remembering traumatic events you have experienced is not easy. So, why would anyone want to think about their traumatic experience(s)? The premise of CPT is that sometimes people get *stuck* in PTSD but that it's possible to get *unstuck* and recover from the effects of trauma. As you'll read later, people get stuck in PTSD when a traumatic experience has not been fully processed, and so the symptoms keep popping up in their life today. So, to address the ongoing symptoms, it's helpful to figure out where you got stuck in your recovery from the event and face the trauma so that it no longer has a hold on you and your life.

In the past, you may have thought about the trauma without feeling any sense of resolution, or feeling like you were not making any progress in recovering. This book will guide you step-by-step through concepts and strategies to address your traumatic experiences in a way that can help you process what you have been through and move toward recovery. If you're willing to put in the work, the tools in this book can help you figure out where you have gotten stuck and how to move forward.

Getting unstuck means doing the opposite of what you may have been doing in the past: trying to ignore the memory of the event or avoiding the triggers that bring up the memories. While those strategies might seem to work in the short run, in the long run you've probably found that they keep you stuck. Instead we'll ask you to think about what you have been saying to yourself about the traumatic events and to examine your automatic thoughts to see if they are factually correct and if they are really helping you in your recovery. When you change what you are saying to yourself to be more balanced and factual, your emotions will change and you'll be able to move forward in your recovery. You may find yourself feeling other emotions that are universal after a trauma and flow naturally from the event (like sadness or disgust), but unlike the feelings you have when you are stuck in your recovery, these feelings will run their course fairly quickly and eventually subside.

Reynaldo had been experiencing PTSD symptoms since one of his friends was shot and killed when he was a young adult. He was supposed to be with his friend that night, but had gotten called into work. After it happened, people asked why he hadn't tried to stop his friend from going to such a dangerous part of town, and Reynaldo felt a lot of guilt. His parents told him not to dwell on what had happened. When he tried to talk with his sister about his feelings after the funeral, she reacted angrily and told him it was time to move on. Reynaldo started to try to push the thoughts and feelings away. He avoided places where he had spent time with friends. When the memories were hard to control, he would drink or smoke marijuana to try to get rid of them. But they kept coming up, even a few years after the event. Mostly, when he thought of what happened, he felt guilty, ashamed, and angry at himself. These feelings didn't go away on their own.

Reynaldo began CPT and started to face his trauma. He did the CPT exercises when he noticed thoughts that were keeping him stuck, including identifying and examining some of the thoughts that had been making him feel guilty, like thinking "I should have been there" or "I could have prevented it." Reynaldo started looking at the evidence for these beliefs and considered whether these thoughts were realistic. As his guilt and anger at himself decreased, he noticed that he was starting to feel grief and anger at the person who had shot his friend, which made sense. At first, the emotions were pretty strong. Reynaldo would let himself cry when he felt sad, but sometimes, such as when he was at work when they came up, he would acknowledge the sadness, take a break and listen to some music, and then get back to work. Soon he noticed that the feelings of grief and sadness were less intense, and he began to also have some happy memories of his friend. The memory of the trauma was still there, but it didn't have the same power over him that it once had.

We're so glad you have found your way to this book. In the next chapter, you will learn more about how you may have gotten stuck in PTSD and how to get unstuck using the tools in this book.

2

How PTSD Keeps You Stuck

The word *trauma* can mean different things to different people. In this book, when we use the word *trauma,* we are referring to a particular type of event.

What Is a Traumatic Event?

When diagnosing PTSD, a traumatic event is defined as one that involves "actual or threatened death, serious injury, or sexual violence" that a person experiences, witnesses directly, or is indirectly exposed to through a close family member or loved one's experience (for example, learning that a close family member or friend died violently or accidentally). Some examples of potentially traumatic events are:

- Rape, sexual abuse, or any other unwanted sexual experience
- Physical assault, such as physical abuse or intimate partner violence
- The murder, drug overdose, or suicide of a loved one
- Combat, such as experiencing or witnessing injury or death
- Serious accidents, such as a motor vehicle accident or an accident at work
- Events that police, firefighters, or other first responders are exposed to involving witnessing severe injury or death
- Natural disasters, such as fires, tornadoes, or hurricanes
- School shootings or other mass violence events
- Race-based trauma
- Experiencing war or violence and being forced to leave one's country or family behind due to danger (war refugee)

Other events, such as a divorce, loss of an aging relative by natural causes, loss of a job, or the end of an important relationship, can be extremely stressful and emotionally difficult. You may find yourself distracted, preoccupied, and very sad or angry about these things.

However, what distinguishes these stressful events from trauma is whether they involved an immediate threat to life or physical injury or violation. Some of the tools and exercises in this book can be helpful for these other stressful experiences, but CPT was designed and tested for PTSD, so we know less about how well it works for other stressors than we do for traumatic events.

Getting Stuck

If a traumatic event is severe enough, almost everyone will experience symptoms of PTSD for at least a while. Your brain needs to process the experience, and traumatic events are hard to sort out, especially if they contradict prior beliefs and expectations about how you think the world should work (more on that later). For many people, the symptoms of PTSD start during or almost immediately after the event is over. For others, the symptoms may show up later, once they are in a safer situation or when something else stressful happens that brings back the memories from the past.

Some of the symptoms of PTSD include intrusive, unwanted images or thoughts of the event popping into your mind, such as when you are reminded of the event, tired, or feeling vulnerable. This is different from thinking about it on purpose. The memories or images can occur when you are awake as flashes of the event or when you are asleep as nightmares. These images are often accompanied by strong emotional reactions that may include fear, guilt, shame, anger, sadness, or horror. Also common are strong startle responses; constantly looking around for danger (hypervigilance); problems with sleep or concentration; or reactive behaviors, like irritable or reckless behavior or perhaps self-harm.

To try to cope with these distressing images, emotions, and physical reactions, people often try avoiding them. There are generally two kinds of avoidance: trying to escape or avoid internal experiences, such as thoughts or emotions; and trying to escape or avoid external reminders of traumatic events, such as people, places, or situations that remind you of the trauma or feel more dangerous since the trauma. There are endless ways that people avoid. Some people avoid certain locations or types of people. Some try to push all memories of the events out of their head by staying as busy as possible. Some people avoid by eating too much (or not enough or purging) or drinking or using drugs. People will try almost anything to avoid the memories and emotions of the traumatic event. It makes sense why someone would want to avoid memories or reminders of the trauma, but as it turns out, avoiding the trauma is part of what keeps people stuck in PTSD.

Cynthia had been abused since childhood, and avoidance had become her main coping style. As a child growing up in an unsafe home environment, she didn't have the option to process her traumatic events while they were happening. As she got older, she boxed up her memories and tried not to think about the past. During adolescence her avoidance also took the form of self-harm—scratching her arms—when memories emerged, particularly after being raped. She felt like she could distract herself from the memories and emotions by inflicting pain on herself. When she first started working through her trauma, she avoided doing the activities initially because she was afraid that if she let her memories and emotions out, they would never stop and would overwhelm her. Fortunately, she had a friend who encouraged her to keep at it and shared her own experience with trauma recovery. With her friend's encouragement and checking in on her frequently, Cynthia was able to continue to process her trauma and began to feel less afraid of her memories after looking at them using the worksheets.

You may have already noticed that the natural tendency to try to avoid trauma memories often has the unintended effect of making the memories pop up more. The intrusive trauma memories and nightmares might be an indication that your mind is still trying to make sense of what happened. It's unlikely that you'll adequately process your trauma if you're working hard at avoiding, so over time the symptoms continue.

Of course, people don't avoid because they want to be stuck with PTSD symptoms. Many people didn't have the support or resources after the trauma that would have allowed them to think about and process their experience. Or they may have had to just survive and get through that period of time, and it was not realistic to stop and make sense of the trauma then or feel their emotions. Over time, not thinking about the trauma can become a habit, and the event may continue to go unprocessed, leading to ongoing symptoms. People may have even suggested that you try to take your mind off it, like "Just forget about it. Put it behind you. Focus on something else." While that logic may work for less significant events, just not thinking about it doesn't work as well for traumatic events (which become the elephant in the room).

The good news is, it's never too late to deal with your trauma and get back on the road to recovery. The fact that you are reading this suggests that you are ready to take that step.

Measuring Your PTSD Symptoms

The first step in assessing your PTSD symptoms is determining whether you have experienced a traumatic event. Did you experience a life-threatening event, serious injury, or sexual violation? It could have been something you experienced directly, witnessed, or learned about happening to someone close. Following are some examples of traumatic experiences. Check off any that have happened to you and use the "other trauma" box if you experienced a trauma that isn't listed here. (Please don't be afraid to write in this book even though you might be tempted to just read the book and not fill out the forms—writing will make a big difference in how helpful the exercises are.)

❑ Physical assault (including by a family member)

❑ Sexual assault (or any unwanted sexual experience)

❑ Feeling like your life was in danger or that you were going to be seriously hurt (including race-based trauma and stalking)

❑ Military combat or living in a war zone

❑ Childhood physical or sexual abuse

❑ Accident

❑ Natural disaster

❑ Accidental or violent death of a loved one

❑ Witnessing or experiencing violence in your community or home country

❑ Witnessing or experiencing the aftermath of a trauma through your work (for example, a first responder being exposed to crime scenes)

❑ Other trauma: _____

Many people have experienced more than one traumatic event in their lives. In working on PTSD symptoms, though, it's important to identify a place to start, even if you eventually work through more than one event. It can help to make a timeline of what's happened to you before you start to work on your PTSD symptoms. Below is an example of a timeline for Isabel. Isabel is like many individuals we have worked with in that she has experienced more than one traumatic event, and she had trouble deciding where to start when working on her PTSD. The items with the brackets represent ongoing, repeated traumas, and the single lines represent individual events.

Use the line at the bottom of this page to make a timeline of the traumatic events you have experienced. Notice from Isabel's example that you don't need to go into detail—just a few words to identify the type of experience will do. You can skip this step if there is one traumatic experience that you know was much more difficult or severe than the others. That event will be your starting point.

Isabel's Traumatic Events Timeline

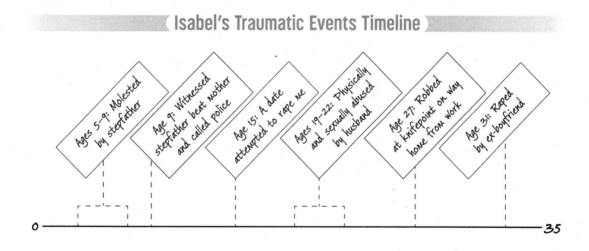

Age 0 _____ Now

As you begin to work through this book, you'll choose one traumatic event *as a starting point*—what we call your *index event*—but over time you can apply what you're learning to other traumas you have faced. The trauma to start with should be the one that haunts you the most. Until you deal with that one, you won't see much change in your PTSD symptoms because that's the one that is keeping you stuck the most. If it isn't easy to identify a trauma that's the "worst" because all traumas are by nature terrible and can have a profound impact on you, you could choose the first one you remember experiencing or the one that you have the most difficult memories of. Often it's the trauma that you most want to avoid thinking about that is the most important place to start. Choose the one that you think you might have the most PTSD symptoms around. Here are some questions to consider:

- How did you react as you made your timeline? Was one trauma harder to think about than others? The worst event is often the one that's hardest to think or talk about.

- Was there something that happened to you personally? Often the closer to you a trauma occurred (happening to you personally versus witnessing or learning about a trauma happening to someone else), the more likely it is to be your index event.

- Was there an event that happened to you in childhood that you have tried to bury in your mind? Your index event may not be the most recent event. You may have one that you are more comfortable talking about, but which is the event that you really push away and try not to deal with?

- All else being equal, is there an event that you have the most guilt, shame, or self-blame about?

If the trauma you experienced was ongoing, or a series of events, it's also helpful to choose the worst part of it to focus on, such as one particular instance. If you aren't sure which is the worst instance, consider the following questions:

- Which event in the series do you have the most intrusive symptoms about, like nightmares or unwanted memories popping up?

- Is there one instance that triggers the strongest emotions, such as guilt, shame, or fear?

- Is there one instance that you avoid thinking about the most?

- Which one do you want to think or talk about the least?

Sometimes the worst event is one that was the most dangerous or severe—like the worst instance of physical abuse you experienced or the mortar attack that hit closest to you where you were the most injured or the most people died. Other times an instance might haunt you more because of the circumstances or meaning. For example, we've worked with people who have experienced years of regular physical abuse by a partner but chose a specific incident, such as when they were severely assaulted while pregnant. We've also worked with people who were sexually abused for years but chose the worst event as the time it happened after they finally told someone it was going on, or a time when, for some reason, they blamed themselves for it more than the perpetrator, such as when they were older and thought they "should have known better." There may be one day or a single event that stands out above all others. It could be a moment when you thought you were going to die, or that saying "No" made no difference, or that other people were in danger and you couldn't help them.

In Isabel's case, she realized that the first series of traumatic events haunted her the most and shaped the way she responded to later events. She felt shame and guilt that she had experienced the molestation. She decided to start with a vivid memory of sexual abuse by her stepfather when she was about five or six that caused her to feel a great deal of fear and shame. Over the course of CPT, she began to work on other memories and events too, but only after she worked on that first vivid and most difficult memory. She found that by having worked on that memory first, she was able to take what she had learned and deal more easily with the other events and memories.

Try not to get stuck on the step of picking an event. If all your traumatic events seem equally bad, choose the event you think would be most helpful to focus on, and get started. Or, if all seem equal, choose the first traumatic event that caused PTSD symptoms. Next, using the "index trauma" you've identified, fill in the Baseline PTSD Checklist on pages 14–15 to assess your current PTSD symptoms (or download it from *www.guilford.com/resick2-forms*). This will represent the level of PTSD symptoms you're experiencing before you start using the skills in this book—your baseline. Answer each question with that specific event in mind. The PTSD Checklist is a commonly used measure for assessing the severity of PTSD symptoms. It asks about symptoms you've been having related to a "stressful experience," and by that it means the index event, the worst traumatic experience that is bothering you the most and will be your starting point in this process. If you are having a hard time deciding between two of the numbers on the scale, for example, a 1 or a 2, choose the higher one. Then add up your score on all of the individual items to get your total score.

If you experienced a traumatic event and your total score is 31 or higher, you are experiencing significant symptoms of PTSD. Fortunately, the skills in this book were developed for people just like you. Even patients with very high scores on the Baseline PTSD Checklist have recovered with CPT. If your score is less than 31, you may still have some PTSD symptoms as indicated by your responses to the items, and you may still benefit from the activities in this book. You'll have opportunities to complete the PTSD Checklist repeatedly as you progress through this book so that you can track your symptoms and make sure you are improving. CPT was developed to treat precisely these symptoms, so continue on to the next chapter to learn more about what you'll do in this process to move toward trauma recovery.

Baseline PTSD Checklist

Instructions: This questionnaire asks about problems you may have had after a very stressful experience involving *actual or threatened death*, *serious injury*, or *sexual violence*. It could be something that happened to you directly, something you witnessed, or something you learned happened to a close family member or close friend. Some examples are a *serious accident; fire; disaster,* such as a *hurricane, tornado,* or *earthquake; physical* or *sexual attack* or *abuse; war; homicide;* or *suicide.*

First, please answer a few questions about your *worst event* (the index event that causes the most PTSD symptoms), which for this questionnaire means the event that currently bothers you the most. This could be one of the examples above or some other very stressful experience.

Briefly identify the worst event: _____

_____

How long ago did it happen? _____

Did it involve actual or threatened death, serious injury, or sexual violence?

❑ Yes

❑ No

How did you experience it?

❑ It happened to me directly.

❑ I witnessed it.

❑ I learned about it happening to a close family member or close friend.

❑ I was repeatedly exposed to details about it as part of my job (for example, paramedic, police, military, or other first responder).

❑ Other (please describe): _____

If the event involved the death of a close family member or close friend, was it due to some kind of accident or violence, or was it due to natural causes?

❑ Accident or violence

❑ Natural causes

❑ Not applicable (the event did not involve the death of a close family member or close friend)

(continued)

Instructions: Below is a list of problems that people sometimes have in response to a very stressful experience. Please read each problem carefully, and then circle one of the numbers to the right to indicate how much you have been bothered by that problem *in the past month*.

In the past month, how much were you bothered by:	Not at all	A little bit	Mod- erately	Quite a bit	Extremely
1. Repeated, disturbing, and unwanted memories of the stressful experience?	0	1	2	3	4
2. Repeated, disturbing dreams of the stressful experience?	0	1	2	3	4
3. Suddenly feeling or acting as if the stressful experience were actually happening again (*as if you were actually back there reliving it*)?	0	1	2	3	4
4. Feeling very upset when something reminded you of the stressful experience?	0	1	2	3	4
5. Having strong physical reactions when something reminded you of the stressful experience (*for example, heart pounding, trouble breathing, sweating*)?	0	1	2	3	4
6. Avoiding memories, thoughts, or feelings related to the stressful experience?	0	1	2	3	4
7. Avoiding external reminders of the stressful experience (*for example, people, places, conversations, activities, objects, or situations*)?	0	1	2	3	4
8. Trouble remembering important parts of the stressful experience (not due to head injury or substances)?	0	1	2	3	4
9. Having strong negative beliefs about yourself, other people, or the world (*for example, having thoughts such as I am bad, There is something seriously wrong with me, No one can be trusted, or The world is completely dangerous*)?	0	1	2	3	4
10. Blaming yourself or someone else (who didn't intend the outcome) for the stressful experience or what happened after it?	0	1	2	3	4
11. Having strong negative feelings, such as fear, horror, anger, guilt, or shame?	0	1	2	3	4
12. Loss of interest in activities that you used to enjoy?	0	1	2	3	4
13. Feeling distant or cut off from other people?	0	1	2	3	4
14. Trouble experiencing positive feelings (*for example, being unable to feel happiness or have loving feelings for people close to you*)?	0	1	2	3	4
15. Irritable behavior, angry outbursts, or acting aggressively?	0	1	2	3	4
16. Taking too many risks or doing things that could cause you harm?	0	1	2	3	4
17. Being "super alert" or watchful or on guard?	0	1	2	3	4
18. Feeling jumpy or easily startled?	0	1	2	3	4
19. Having difficulty concentrating?	0	1	2	3	4
20. Trouble falling or staying asleep?	0	1	2	3	4

Add up the total and write it here: _____

(The possible range of scores is 0–80.)

3

Making a Plan to Get Unstuck from PTSD

Now that you've identified whether this book is a good match for the kinds of problems you've been facing, you may be wondering what is involved in the process. This book will help you work with the thoughts that keep you stuck in your PTSD, like what you tell yourself about why the traumatic event happened and what you think the trauma means about you, other people, and the world. Probably most of your thoughts about your trauma are accurate and helpful. However, there may be some things you've been telling yourself that are less helpful or that you haven't really thought about very deeply to make sure they are true. For example, like many people with PTSD, Isabel blamed herself for the molestation she experienced as a child and questioned whether she did something to cause it or didn't do enough to stop it, even if another option wasn't really realistic at the time. Isabel thought she should have tried to fight her stepfather off and shouldn't have "given up" and "let" him molest her. She also thought she should have told someone right after it happened the first time. Like others with PTSD, Isabel got stuck thinking negatively about herself and other people; she thought she was "too damaged" to be loved because of what had happened to her and believed she could never trust anyone again. Thoughts like these can cause negative emotions, like guilt, shame, fear, or anger, and get in the way of living the kind of life you want to live.

If there are any thoughts you've been having about the trauma that keep you stuck, you may need to take time to look carefully at the facts. Using the skills contained in this book, Isabel came to understand that she was very young when she was abused by her stepfather, she had been afraid, and he had told her he would hurt her if she told anyone. As she worked through the exercises, she was able to let go of some of the shame she felt, as she realized that she was a child who had had no control over what happened and that her stepfather was the adult who had made the decision to abuse her. She realized it wasn't fair to herself to think of herself as "damaged" by something she couldn't control. She thought about all of the ways that she was resilient and realized that who she is as a person is defined by much more than those traumatic events that she had experienced. By going back and considering the larger context as Isabel did, you may come to think differently about your role in your traumatic event and what it now means about you and your life generally. If some of your thinking about the trauma changes, your emotions may change as well, and you may notice a sense of relief or a decrease in the intensity of your reactions to traumatic memories. The activities and worksheets in this book will guide you to examine your thoughts to help you make sense of the event.

The skills and concepts in this book can help you get unstuck and moving toward recovery by helping you to:

- Understand PTSD and how avoidance can fuel PTSD symptoms.
- Identify how your thoughts and feelings interact.
- Experience and process your emotions related to traumatic events.
- Identify thoughts that keep you stuck in PTSD.
- Examine these thoughts based on the facts of the situation, including facts that you may have overlooked or forgotten.
- Understand how traumatic events impacted your sense of safety, trust, power/control, esteem, and intimacy.
- Develop more balanced and adaptive ways to think about your traumas, why they happened, and their impact on your life and future.

The ultimate goal is for you to develop specialized new thinking skills that you would not have been taught in school or by your parents and that you can apply not only to past events but to any difficult situations in the future. By learning the series of skills in this book, you'll have the opportunity to gain control over your trauma instead of your trauma having control over you. You can use these skills during your work in this book and long after. People who have completed CPT have noticed decreases in flashbacks and nightmares, startle responses, and avoidance of reminders, as well as better relationships with others and improved self-esteem. About half of the people who have PTSD also have depression, and successfully treating PTSD symptoms has been shown to lead to improvement in depression as well.

How to Use This Book

This book contains the tools that you'll need to process your traumatic experiences. Each section contains new information and skills, as well as practice activities. If you have access to the Internet through a computer, tablet, or phone, there are also videos we refer you to that may further help you understand the skills and concepts, such as how to fill out a specific worksheet. See the box on the next page for specific tips for using the book.

Pacing Your Work

A great thing about using this book is that you can go at your own pace and don't need to schedule appointments with a provider to work toward recovery, and you can do it

Tips for Using This Book

⮐ Try to work on it every day, or at least four or five days a week.

⮐ Pick a good time when you can be free of distractions and spend at least fifteen minutes.

⮐ You can work at your own pace, but we recommend working on roughly one chapter each week.

⮐ Write in this book—don't just "think through" the answers. That way you can go back and see your work, revisit some skills and ideas, and see how far you've come.

⮐ You don't have to practice each exercise until you get it perfect! Each chapter builds on the last, and you'll get to keep practicing as you go. What matters is that you use the exercises to slow down and think through the questions you're asked in each section.

⮐ Remember, developing a new skill takes practice! It might feel awkward at first, but like anything, with practice it gets easier and the new skills may even become new habits.

⮐ Watch out for avoidance! You may find that you don't want to think about the trauma, or you might find other things that you think you need to be doing before you get around to your daily practice. Remember, you are making a commitment to yourself to work on your recovery—and at times that might be hard—but it's worth sticking with it!

anywhere you are. However, it's important for you to remain focused, and it's best to work on it every day.

As you move through the book, you can decide when you have practiced the skills in each chapter enough to move on to the next. We recommend spending no more than one week on each chapter if you are practicing each day. It's important to know that *you don't have to be able to use each skill perfectly,* because the next set of skills will build on the previous ones and allow you to continue practicing. In fact, some people never quite get the hang of some of the skills, but they do the best they can and still recover. That being said, it's important to complete the major practice assignments that are the core of CPT because that's what we know works to help people recover.

Some people move through the process quickly, such as in a few weeks, while others might work through one section each week and take a few months to complete the process. Both of these paces have been tested for CPT with a therapist and shown to work, so you can choose whichever pace works best for you. What pace would make the most sense for you and your life?

Setting goals for how you'll work through this book can also help you make steady progress. But even if you skip a day—just jump back in the next day.

What time of day will you do the practice? _____

How will you make sure there are few or no distractions when you work on it, and how will you remember to practice?

_____

_____

_____

_____

People sometimes put reminders on their phone or on their calendars. Other people get into the habit of doing the work at the same time every day, like when they are on a break at work or after dinner before they watch television. How will you make sure that you prioritize some practice every day?

Use the calendar on the next page to map out your plan or download it from *www. guilford.com/resick2-forms*.

Follow these instructions for using the calendar:

- First, fill in the calendar days starting with the current month.

- Next, mark on the calendar how much time you'll spend working through the skills in this book each day for the weeks ahead. For example, you might plan to spend 15–20 minutes per day on most days, but 5–10 minutes per day during a week you know you'll be busy at work or school. Assuming you complete all chapters and do a little each day, you might complete one chapter per week and finish in 12 weeks. We encourage you to keep a steady pace because we do not have any data that working on the skills less than once a week is effective.

- Set a date you hope to be done with CPT that you can look forward to based on your plan. This might help you later because you can remind yourself that if you keep working at it, you can stay on track with your goal.

- Schedule or plan some rewards for yourself after you complete each section. It's important to acknowledge the hard work that you're doing.

Take a moment to write down your schedule for working regularly through this book. You may also want to block off some time or set reminders in an electronic calendar if you use one.

Put a sticky note on the next page (or keep handy your printed copy) with your completed calendar, or use some other bookmark to make it easy to refer back to it and continue to track your progress. Of course, your plan may not work out exactly this way, and that's OK. The point is to have a plan for when you will get the work done so that you can keep moving toward recovery. If you deviate from your plan, no problem. Get back to the work as soon as possible and alter your plan as needed.

CPT Planning Calendar

Month: _____

Sunday	Monday	Tuesday	Wednesday	Thursday	Friday	Saturday

Month: _____

Sunday	Monday	Tuesday	Wednesday	Thursday	Friday	Saturday

Month: _____

Sunday	Monday	Tuesday	Wednesday	Thursday	Friday	Saturday

Month: _____

Sunday	Monday	Tuesday	Wednesday	Thursday	Friday	Saturday

As you progress through the book, you'll monitor your symptoms and determine when you no longer need to continue. Consider the following:

- Each week or chapter, you'll monitor your progress using the PTSD Checklist. If you start feeling better and are satisfied with your progress, you can double-check your symptom levels to see if your scores have dropped to a non-PTSD level.

- Scores below 20 are indicative of a good outcome. A reduction of 10 points or more is also considered a significant amount of symptom change. But ultimately you get to decide when you have seen the benefits you need to move forward in your life.

- If you decide to stop before completing all of the chapters, then you can go to the final chapters to wrap up your work. You'll have an opportunity to reflect on your progress and ensure you have made the changes that you want and notice anything else you want to keep working on in the future.

Note: *If you are working with a therapist or decide you could benefit from working with one, you and your therapist will decide when to meet, such as once or twice per week.* You should let the therapist know that you have this book and share your work with them. If you work with a CPT therapist, the worksheets and handouts they give you may look somewhat different, but the concepts are the same. You can use the worksheets and assignments supplied by a CPT-trained therapist or share this book with a non-CPT therapist.

The Importance of Practice

Research has shown that people who complete more practice activities during PTSD treatment get greater improvements in their symptoms. Therefore, it is very important that you complete the activities in this book to get the full benefit.

Why practice? To learn any new skill, whether it's tying your shoe, driving a car, learning to cook, excelling at a sport, or learning a language, you must practice repeatedly until it becomes a habit. If you have been thinking one way ever since your traumatic events began, then it takes practice to learn how to examine and possibly change what you have been saying automatically.

The more work you put in, the more likely you are to benefit, and the sooner you start, the sooner you can start feeling better. We encourage you to do your best to overcome the symptoms of avoidance and commit to doing the activities long enough to see results.

Common Questions before Starting

What should I do if something stressful happens in my life?

Stressful events, good or bad, are part of life and not a reason to quit working on your PTSD. Even if you experience a stressful event, it can still be helpful to keep working on your trauma. After all, it will be a lot easier to manage day-to-day stress once you have recovered from PTSD. However, if the stressful experience is very severe (like the death of a loved one, loss of a job or home, or a sudden health problem), you may need to take a short break to allow yourself to manage the crisis and process your emotions about that event. If you can, use some of the skills you are learning in this book to examine your thoughts and feelings about the stressor. The skills that you are learning here can be applied to other events in your life and can help you avoid falling into old ways of thinking that are related to your PTSD. As soon as you can, come back to the activities here to keep working on your PTSD.

What should I do if my PTSD starts to feel worse?

Sometimes when people stop avoiding (which is actually a PTSD symptom decrease!), other symptoms might increase temporarily, like feeling more emotions or having nightmares. You are allowing yourself to remember the trauma because you are not pushing it away, and that's a good thing. Doing so gives you the chance to process what happened and move toward recovery. Remind yourself that it's a memory and that the event is over. Avoidance kept the PTSD going all this time, and now you're stopping and facing those memories, thoughts, and emotions. By the end of Chapter 8, if you do the practice assignments thoughtfully and regularly, you may notice that you are beginning to feel better. But don't worry if it takes a little longer. Some people notice it takes more time, and we'll have troubleshooting suggestions along the way.

Make sure to give the program a chance to work, and don't give up before you have an opportunity to benefit. Some people take longer than others until something eventually clicks and they start seeing symptom improvement. You may find that it's helpful to ask family and friends to support you while you do this work (see the handout "Supporting Your Loved One During CPT" in the Appendix) and to let them know that you may be experiencing some emotional ups and downs. If they see that, they can encourage you to stick with it. It won't be helpful if they tell you to stop doing the work (unless they see that you are at risk of harming yourself or engaging in other unhealthy coping behaviors, in which case it will be important to get some professional help). Instead, they can encourage you to take care of yourself and to do some things you enjoy as well.

See the box on the facing page if you are experiencing thoughts about suicide.

What if I get stuck?

As you go through this process, you'll learn many new skills. It's not expected that you'll "master" every concept right away. Even if you find something challenging or difficult to understand, this book will guide you to continue to build your skills as you move along in the program. It's important not to feel like you have to do everything "perfectly" to move on. It's much more important to stick with it and keep going.

If you have a hard time understanding a concept or worksheet, you can use the videos that are suggested throughout the book to help increase your understanding. There are also troubleshooting guides and example worksheets after each section and additional sources of help in the Resources at the end of this book. However, if you are working on your own and feel like you are still stuck, consider finding a therapist to help.

A Few Words about Suicidal Thoughts and Feelings

Many people suffering from PTSD have thoughts about hurting or killing themselves at some point. If you are in danger of hurting yourself and feeling like you can't keep yourself safe, it's important to reach out for help right away. In the United States, you can contact the National Suicide Prevention Lifeline (call or text 988) or go online to *www.988lifeline.org* to chat. You can also text HOME to 741741 to contact the Crisis Text Line, or go to a hospital. (Hotlines for other English-speaking countries can be found in the Resources.)

CPT is very effective, but it's important that you do not harm yourself before you give the skills a chance to work. Research has shown that people who complete CPT experience decreases in suicidal thinking. Once you are feeling better, you may find that you're looking forward to your life as you continue in your recovery and that urges to die decrease. In the meantime, reaching out for help and developing a suicide prevention safety plan, such as the one found in the PTSD Coach mobile app (*www.ptsd.va.gov/appvid/mobile/ptsdcoach_app.asp*), can help you get the support you need as you work on your recovery.

Goal Setting: What Are You Working Toward?

Before you begin working through the rest of this book, it can help to take a step back and remind yourself of the reasons you've decided to work on your PTSD. What made you decide to take this step? Some people decide that they need to work on their PTSD because it interferes with something important to them, like their relationships with family, their work, or their ability to do things they enjoy without experiencing intense feelings or reminders.

What are some of your goals and some of your reasons to work on your PTSD?

_____

_____

_____

_____

How will you know if you're starting to feel better—what would you like to change as you recover from PTSD?

_____

_____

_____

_____

Assessing Your Progress

Just as you filled out the Baseline PTSD Checklist to assess your current PTSD symptoms, we recommend filling out a new PTSD Checklist each week while you are completing this book, kind of like taking your temperature each time you go to the doctor, to see how your symptoms change. This way you can track your progress and make sure you are moving toward recovery. We have included a PTSD Checklist at the end of each chapter for you to assess where you are with your symptoms. You don't need to take it more than once a week if you are moving quickly through the book. Be sure to keep rating your PTSD symptoms on the same traumatic event, your index trauma, each week. You can use the Graph for Tracking Your Weekly Scores below (or print one out from *www.guilford.com/resick2-forms*) to mark your progress. Dog-ear this page, put a sticky note on it, or keep handy your printed copy so you can refer back to it to track your progress each week.

Each week, mark your total score on the graph. Make a dot where the week number you are on matches your score on the left-hand side. You can start by putting your first score

Graph for Tracking Your Weekly Scores

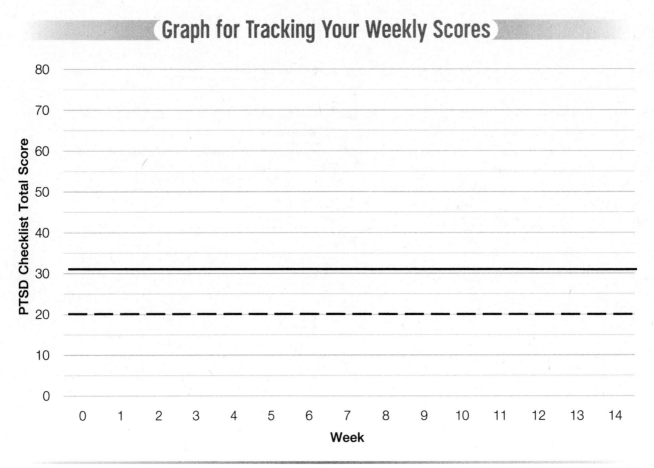

from your Baseline PTSD Checklist on pages 14–15 down for Week 0. As you add more scores over the weeks ahead, connect each dot to your last dot to track whether your scores are decreasing. Consider the following:

- Scores of 31 or more (the solid line) indicate you probably have PTSD. CPT was originally developed for people who have PTSD. However, you may benefit even if your score is lower to start.

- Track your scores as you continue through the process. Remember, if your score drops below 31, you are starting to look more like someone who no longer has intense PTSD symptoms. If your score drops below 20 (the dashed line), you probably no longer have a clinical level of PTSD, and this is considered a good outcome score. Reductions of 10 or more points also indicate significant improvement.

An example graph for Louis, who completed the program in 11 weeks, is at the bottom of the page.

As you can see, Louis started with significant PTSD symptoms. His symptoms steadily decreased as he went through the program. He ended at a score of 18, which was a substantial reduction from his starting score (more than 10 points).

It's even more important to notice how you are feeling in your life. Are your relationships improving? Are you thinking about new goals you want to achieve? Are you haunted less by the memories of the traumatic events? The goal is not to forget that these events happened, because they are part of your life, but to accept that they happened without currently experiencing overwhelming emotions. You might start thinking "I remember how bad I

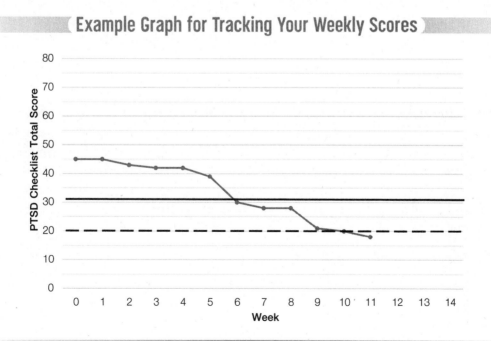

Example Graph for Tracking Your Weekly Scores

used to feel whenever I thought about what happened, but now I can think of it without the urge to run away from the memory."

~~~~~~~~~~ How to Start ~~~~~~~~~~

You've decided this book might be helpful. What should you do now? The best thing you can do is to get started right away with the next chapter. Remember that avoidance is a symptom of PTSD, so don't avoid or procrastinate—start today if you can. The next chapter (Chapter 4) covers more education about PTSD and explains the concepts you'll need to move through the rest of the book. You'll learn more about PTSD, why people get stuck with it, and how you can get unstuck from it by using the approaches in this book. You'll also have an opportunity to reflect on how symptoms of PTSD have affected your life.

Anticipating Roadblocks

Are you nervous or hesitant about getting started? There are many common roadblocks people face as they begin to consider working on their trauma. It's common for people to feel stuck or hesitant even before they begin. These might even be forms of avoidance. Here are some common roadblocks that might get in the way of starting this process, or being as successful as possible with it, and some points to consider for each.

I'm afraid of reliving my trauma.

Thinking or writing about your trauma is not the same thing as "reliving" or "reexperiencing" it. For most people working on their PTSD, the trauma is in the past and over. Although you may sometimes feel like the memories are so vivid that it's like it's still happening, if the trauma is in the past, you are safe from it now. Although it may bring up very unpleasant emotions, *it's not dangerous to think about past traumas*. The memories are already in your mind, so this work involves *acknowledging what is already there,* but *it does not create any new trauma*.

Doing this work may also help you recognize the difference between experiencing the trauma and remembering it, and give you more confidence in your ability to manage your emotional reactions. You may also gain a greater sense of control over your trauma memories versus feeling like the memories control you. In the past, you may have thought about the trauma and just felt worse. However, this book will help you think about your trauma in a systematic, therapeutic way to help you get unstuck.

I'm not sure which trauma to start with.

Previously we talked about identifying an index event to start with, but it's common for this to be a difficult step. Maybe you skipped over that, or maybe you've found yourself questioning if you've really picked the best event to start with. Sometimes people get so focused on choosing the "right" event that they end up avoiding doing the work and don't benefit as much. As a reminder, it's best to start with the trauma that is most at the heart of your PTSD, the one that is haunting you the most. If you don't know which one that is, look back over the Baseline PTSD Checklist you completed earlier (pages 14–15), which includes the symptoms of PTSD, and ask yourself which event causes most of these symptoms. If they all seem equally bad, you could pick the one that you have the most guilt or self-blame over or the one that came first. Often it is the one that you want to think about least that would be most beneficial to work on first.

Also, sometimes people feel bad for choosing one trauma over another. For example, you might feel guilty not picking a trauma where someone close to you was killed. In that case, you could ask yourself what that person would want for you. Would they want you to feel guilty, or would they want you to work on the trauma that is causing you the most PTSD so you can get better? Overall, it's important not to get too hung up on which one to start with at the expense of getting going with the steps that will help you start feeling better. So, pick the one you think would be most helpful to work on and get started with that one, and you can address the other traumas later on in the process.

Am I ready? Maybe I should wait until I have more time to do this right.

It's definitely important to make sure you have time to practice the skills in this book. However, we would caution against waiting for the "perfect" time. Life is busy! Instead, see if you can find even fifteen minutes per day when you can practice. For example, you could do it while waiting for dinner to cook, during your lunch break, or while your kids do their homework or just after they go to bed. By doing a little each day, you can continue to make progress on your PTSD. Similarly, some people feel like they have to do the work "exactly right" or read and understand every single word in this book to benefit. Thinking that way often keeps people from doing *any* work, and that's definitely not helpful! If you did it "perfectly" (whatever that means), you probably wouldn't really be feeling your emotions or connecting to your experience. It's OK for this process to be messy and disorganized because that's how trauma memories are in the beginning. Just do your best, get started so that you can begin feeling better, and stick with it!

It's up to you to decide if this program is right for you, but it's also worth considering what is "ready." There may never be a perfect time to work on your traumas. Perhaps another question to consider is whether you are *willing* to do this. If this really worked well and you were able to get relief from your PTSD, would it be worth it to put in the hard work now? If so, we look forward to guiding you as you embark on this process.

Maybe I'll just read this book, but not write anything down. Writing down what happened or my thoughts about it would make it real.

This is something we have heard before, and we would offer as food for thought that the trauma is already real. It happened, and you continue to have memories about it at times that you may not be able to predict. Choosing when to work on it already takes some power from the memories, because instead of the memories, thoughts, and emotions "coming after you" at unpredictable times, you go after the memories at a time that works for you, and with a plan for how to deal with them. It's also real that you have symptoms of PTSD and experience strong emotions and memories. What may or may not be true, however, is what you've been telling yourself about the event, such as that it was your fault or that you could have prevented it somehow. That's what the activities in this book will help you examine. It's important that you fully participate to get the most out of this process, and that means writing in the book. Simply reading through this book may or may not help you with your PTSD—however, we know *CPT can work when clients do the activities and practice the skills.* If you're really having a hard time writing things down, try starting by writing in pencil, which may feel less permanent. Some people also worry about writing because they are afraid what someone might think or do if they saw it. Keeping this book in a private place is important. Some people we have worked with have kept their book in the trunk of their car or in a locker at work, at school, or at the gym. If you prefer, you can download the worksheets from *www.guilford.com/resick2-forms* and work on them outside of this book.

It's great that you have found your way to this book, and you should be proud for taking this step. Dealing with trauma is not easy, but by using the skills you will learn here, recovery is possible. So let's get started—turn to Chapter 4 and begin your journey getting unstuck from PTSD.

Part II

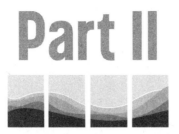

Identifying Where You Are Stuck

The first step in this process is to figure out where you are stuck so that you can work on getting unstuck. In the next few chapters, you'll learn more about what PTSD is and reflect on what PTSD looks like in your life. Then you'll complete an activity to help you identify the specific thoughts that may be getting in the way of your trauma recovery. After that, you'll learn a set of skills to notice the connection between situations, thoughts, and emotions. Through these exercises, you'll likely start to become more aware of what you've been saying to yourself about your trauma and life since then, and how certain thoughts might be fueling some of the emotions you are feeling day-to-day. After completing this section of the book, you'll have your road map for the course ahead and be able to start processing your traumatic experience.

Introduction to PTSD and Trauma Recovery

A basic part of recovering from PTSD is understanding what it is and why you may have it. In this chapter you'll learn more about what PTSD is, why people get stuck in it, and how to get unstuck from it by using this book. You'll also have the chance to reflect on how PTSD looks in your life. Before or after you read this, you may find it helpful to watch the National Center for PTSD whiteboard video *What Is PTSD?* (*https://bit.ly/3zsRvTL*).

PTSD Symptoms

The symptoms of PTSD fall into clusters, or groups of symptoms. The first cluster involves the memory of the event **intruding** on your life today in some way (**intrusive symptoms**). In other words, you are not trying to think about it—the memory just comes to you and might be an image or possibly sounds or smells of the traumatic event(s). It's different from thinking about something on purpose. You might experience intrusive memories that suddenly pop into your mind. You might have the intrusive memories when there is something that reminds you of the event. For example, for some people, anniversaries of the event (or season, weather, or day of the week) bring more intrusive memories. You might notice that when you're in certain places, or when you hear, see, feel, or smell certain things, the memories come up more. You may also experience intrusive memories when there is nothing there to remind you of the trauma. Common times to have these memories push through are when you are falling asleep, relaxing, not feeling well, or bored. These reminders and intrusions may also lead you to feel negative emotions or experience physical changes in your body. You also might have nightmares about the event or other scary dreams, or you might experience flashbacks when you act or feel as if the incident is happening again right now. While many people worry that these experiences mean they are "going crazy," it's common to have intrusive symptoms after a traumatic event. It's your mind's way of trying to process something very extreme and out of the ordinary that happened to you. As you work through the skills in this book and begin to recover, you'll likely notice that you have fewer of these experiences and that even when you do notice reminders, you feel and begin to react to them differently.

Can you write down some examples of these intrusive symptoms that you currently experience?

_____

_____

_____

_____

Another set of symptoms involve **arousal or reactivity**. Arousal refers to how activated your body and mind are. People with PTSD tend to be more keyed up and on edge. When you are reminded of a traumatic event or you experience memories, nightmares, or flash-backs, these can trigger the arousal symptoms cluster. You may notice problems falling or staying asleep, feeling irritable or having angry outbursts, having a hard time concentrating, or experiencing startle reactions like jumping at noises or when someone walks up behind you. You may feel on guard or like you're looking over your shoulder even when there is no reason to. Some people also engage in reckless or self-destructive behavior, like driving too fast or taking risks in other ways.

Which of these arousal and reactivity symptoms do you experience?

_____

_____

_____

_____

A third set of symptoms involves **changes in your mood and the way you think about things** as a result of the trauma. You might find that your mood is mostly negative and that you often feel guilt, shame, anger, fear, and/or sadness. Sometimes people lose interest in doing things they used to enjoy. You may find it hard to experience positive emotions, and you may feel numb and cut off from the world around you. Some people describe a feeling like looking through a window at everyone else living their lives and enjoying themselves but not being able to really connect with them. Have you had numbing or a lack of positive feelings?

_____

When you experience emotions, what are they?

_____

_____

_____

_____

If you experience anger, who is it directed at: yourself or others?

_____

Sometimes people also have trouble remembering all or part of the event. This might be because they have avoided thinking about it for so long. The way you think about things may have also changed since the trauma. You may find that you think about yourself, others, and the world differently, maybe in a much more negative way. How has your thinking changed as a result of the trauma(s)?

_____

_____

_____

_____

After experiencing traumatic events, many people blame themselves or other people for not being able to stop the traumatic event or prevent the trauma from happening, even if that wasn't realistic at the time. Do you find that you blame yourself for the trauma? In what ways might you be taking on too much of the blame?

_____

_____

_____

_____

Other people may know that they did not cause the traumatic event, but they feel angry with and blame other people involved for some aspect of what happened, even if those people didn't intend the trauma to happen either. Does this happen for you? Who do you blame or feel angry toward?

_____

_____

_____

_____

The fourth set of symptoms involves **avoiding** reminders of the event. When you have such strong and painful feelings in reaction to reminders, it's natural to want to push them away or to avoid anything that will remind you of what happened. After all, who would

---

Avoidance Alert!

Avoidance has many faces and may be hard to pick out because it is such a habit. Avoidance isn't as noticeable as flashbacks or panic attacks. You may say, "I don't like to go to parties or eat in restaurants." Did you like them before the traumatic event? If so, it may be avoidance. There are as many types of avoidance as there are people, and you need to keep a close eye out for them. Being angry or aggressive can be an effective form of avoidance because it pushes people away. But what is the cost of that? Using alcohol to get to sleep faster or without having nightmares has short-term gains but could end in dependency or poorer sleep. Overeating or purging can be associated with avoidance of emotions. Some forms of avoidance are very subtle, like thinking "I don't have time to do this because I am just so busy." Did you fill up your life with so many activities that you don't have space to think? Putting this book in a drawer where you won't see it is also avoidance. Even telling jokes as a form of deflection could be avoidance. Many forms of avoidance may have developed outside of your awareness, but they serve a similar function. An example is headaches or other physical pains. A headache may distract you when you are reminded of your trauma memory. You may be afraid that thinking about your trauma will give you a headache. The other way to look at it is that, if you are having headaches anyway, why not do the work and see if they improve? So, why is all this important? Because avoidance is the driver for the continuation of PTSD. As long as you avoid your trauma memories you won't have the opportunity to process the experience, think about it any differently, and let your emotions run their course. Your brain keeps bringing up the topic. Instead of fighting your brain, you need to stand and face your memories, which means you need to work hard to notice and stop avoidance.

---

want to walk around feeling angry, scared, guilty, or sad all the time? So, you might find yourself avoiding places or people who remind you of your traumatic experience. Some people avoid watching certain television programs or turn off the TV when something comes on that reminds them of their trauma. Some people avoid reading the newspaper or watching the news. There might be certain sights, sounds, or smells that you find yourself avoiding or escaping from because they remind you of the event. You might also avoid thinking about the event and letting yourself feel your feelings about it. For some people, that means drinking or staying busy so as not to have time to think about the trauma. Not practicing the skills in this book or deciding not to work on the most difficult traumatic event would also be examples of avoidance (see the box above for more on the different faces of avoidance).

In what ways do you avoid?

_____

_____

_____

_____

How PTSD Develops

The first three symptom clusters described earlier are common for a month or so after a traumatic event. After a trauma, people experience intrusive symptoms, arousal and reactivity symptoms, and negative thoughts and emotions. These reactions trigger one another—so if you have an intrusive memory, it can lead your thoughts and feelings to spiral, and you may notice that you have physical reactions, too. For some people, these symptoms and reactions decrease over time and they experience trauma recovery. We know from decades of research on trauma recovery that those who experience recovery are those who have had an opportunity to think about the trauma and feel their emotions without avoiding. When people have the opportunity to process their thoughts, feelings, and reactions, the strong emotions and physical responses decrease over time and eventually disconnect from each other. Eventually the memory of the trauma doesn't provoke such strong reactions. This is what this book is designed to help you do.

People who go on to develop PTSD do not recover in the same way. Something happens that disrupts the process of recovery, and you get stuck with the symptoms long term. It turns out that the culprit is not having a chance to process the experience, which can happen when there is avoidance. In the beginning, avoidance may be unintentional or out of your control. You may not have had the opportunity to talk to others about your experience or feel emotions. You may have had to just keep going and get through that period of time, and so you may have been forced to push the memories and emotions away. This can happen if the people around you weren't supportive or if you just needed to survive or go on to the next thing after the trauma and couldn't take time to really process what was happening. For example, people in combat may not have time to process the loss of a fellow service member because they may have had to just move on to the next mission. Or if you lived in an abusive household, you may have had to just keep your head down and try to stay safe until you were away from the abusive individuals. But over time, avoidance can take over and may become the norm, and this prevents the other symptoms from changing. After the trauma, when you finally do have time or support to deal with it, you may just want to try to move forward and not look back. However, avoidance stops the adjustment process. The problem is that until you really process it, it won't go away (see the diagram on the next page).

Also, avoidance works in the short term—you might feel relief when you get away from a reminder or think about something more positive—so it's tempting to avoid when emotions are strong and thoughts are disturbing. The problem is that avoidance doesn't work well over the long term. It doesn't fix the PTSD symptoms. The strategies people use to avoid can also lead to other serious problems, such as substance use problems and other addictive behaviors, aggression, depression, and so forth. It can also lead to problems in your relationships because you may find yourself spending less time with people in your life.

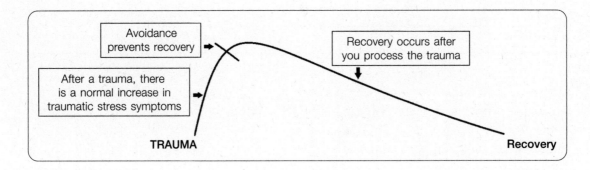

What downsides or consequences of avoidance have you noticed in your own life?

_____

_____

_____

_____

The goal of CPT is to stop the avoidance behaviors and help you start processing your thoughts and feelings in a way that you haven't been able to up until now. Eventually, as you do this work, the traumatic memory will lose the power to send you spiraling into such a bad place. You'll get to a point where you remember how awful the event was and how you felt—but you won't actually experience the same feelings that you did in the moment. The traumatic event and memory will never be erased—they are part of your history—but you can get to a point where they don't dominate your life, your decisions, and your relationships.

Understanding Reactions to Traumatic Events

This section explains reactions to traumatic events in more detail and some of the ways people either recover or get stuck.

Trauma Recovery and the Fight–Flight–Freeze Response

Based on what we just described, it's helpful to think of PTSD as *a problem in recovery*. It's not surprising that you developed some of the symptoms you did, but something got in the way of the natural process of recovery from those symptoms. Your job now is to determine what got in the way and to change it so you can get back on the road to recovery, working to get "unstuck."

You may be having trouble recovering for a variety of reasons. First, there may be factors that date back to the time of the event itself. When people face serious, possibly life-threatening events, they often experience a very strong physical response called the **fight–flight–freeze reaction**. Many people have heard of "fight or flight," but there is also a third possibility: the freeze response. In the fight–flight–freeze reaction, your body undergoes a number of physical changes in response to danger to reduce the risk of serious harm and increase the chance of survival. For example, your body may work to quickly get blood and oxygen out to your hands, feet, and big muscle groups, like your thighs and forearms, so that you can run or fight if you need to. This necessitates reducing function in other parts of the body that are not essential at that moment. After all, you don't need to be thinking about your philosophy of life or digesting dinner if you are in a life-threatening situation. As a result of these physical changes, you might feel like you have been kicked in the gut or are going to faint.

The same thing happens with the freeze response, but in this case your body is trying to reduce both physical and emotional pain. During your trauma, you may have stopped feeling pain or had the sense that the event was happening to someone else, as if you were watching a movie. You might have been completely shut down emotionally or even had shifts in perception like feeling as though you were out of your body or time had slowed down. This is called dissociation. Just like fighting and fleeing, freezing is an automatic response to danger that is adaptive to your survival.

There is another kind of freeze response that happens right at the beginning of a traumatic event. Often when the event starts, it's not clear what's going on. Traumatic events are most often sudden and unexpected, and it can take a moment or two to realize that you are in danger or that something is happening that is out of your control. This is called an *orienting response*. Many people feel ashamed or frustrated at themselves for having this freeze response. However, it's important to remember that the freeze response is hardwired in the brain and is automatic, so it's not your fault if you didn't immediately take action. It was a completely normal response during extreme circumstances.

Different parts of the brain are involved during trauma exposure and later on as part of PTSD. Different brain areas are involved in emotions, thinking, remembering, and putting events into context. Sometimes they form a feedback loop. For example, in the fight–flight–freeze reaction above, when threat is detected, a part of the brain called the *amygdala* causes you to experience strong emotions like fear or anger, and a signal is sent from there to the brainstem to send out messages (neurotransmitters) that alter thinking. As a result, the frontal part of the brain, the thinking part, may have reduced function. The fear can even affect one of the speech centers in the brain. When people describe being speechless in horror, they're not exaggerating. If Broca's area, one of the speech centers, is affected, it may be hard to even talk, which you may have experienced yourself.

Now that the trauma is over and you are working on recovery, it's important to use the frontal cortex of your brain because it's part of that feedback loop. When your thoughts are engaged and you are using words, the message loops back to the amygdala and can reduce how strongly you feel emotions. Completing a worksheet, as you'll learn to do in this book, helps keep the thinking parts of your brain activated, and that helps reduce the runaway emotions. So even if you get to a point where you can use the skills that you learn from this book in your head, there might be times that writing things down on the worksheet can still be helpful in managing strong emotions and thinking more clearly.

Some people do not have the fight–flight–freeze emergency response because they were not in imminent danger during the traumatic event or didn't know they had been in danger until later. For example, if you hear about someone you love having a terrible experience, or witness violence but are not directly threatened yourself, a different part of your brain may react and you may not have the same response. However, you can still get stuck in PTSD due to your thinking and feelings about the traumatic events.

Regardless of whether or not you had a fight–flight–freeze response, after traumatic events people often start to second-guess themselves and think about all of the things they "should" or "could" have done at the time of the traumatic event. They blame themselves for freezing or for not fighting back or doing something to stop, prevent, or save people during the event. But it's important to consider what your state of mind was during the event. Were you taken by surprise? If you are thinking of things you wish you'd done differently, did you have all possible options available to you then? Is it fair to expect that you could make a perfect decision about what to do when your brain was dealing with a trauma in the ways described above? If your trauma occurred when you were much younger, you may have started to blame yourself for not reacting the way you think your current, adult self (or someone else you know) would have reacted. But did you know then what you know now? Do you have skills today that you didn't have back then?

Another thing that can happen when people develop PTSD is that the fight–flight–freeze response or fear experienced during the traumatic event can get paired with other things that were in the environment at the time, such as certain sights, sounds, or smells. Then those cues, which didn't have any particular meaning before, become associated with the trauma or danger more generally and become triggers that lead you to feel strong emotions or think that you are in danger again whenever you come across them. For example, if you get into a car accident on a highway bridge, you might begin to associate all highway bridges, or at least the one you were on, with danger. Then later, when you encounter those triggers, you are likely to have another fight–flight–freeze reaction. Your nervous system senses the trigger, which could be the sight of the bridge, the sound of cars whizzing by you, or even the time of day (like dusk if that's when the accident happened), and then your body reacts as though you are in danger again. If you started to associate bridges with danger, you may start to notice that you feel anxious any time you are approaching a bridge on the highway. These reactions will fade over time if you don't avoid those triggers. If you drive every day along the same route and cross the bridge, and don't avoid other highway bridges, soon you won't associate bridges with danger because most of the time when you cross them you're actually safe.

However, if you avoid triggers and reminder cues, your body and brain won't learn that these are not, in fact, good indications of danger. They don't tell you accurately whether you are actually in danger, so you may have **false alarms** going off frequently. You'll feel the fight–flight–freeze response going off even when you are safe. After a while you won't trust your own senses or judgment about what is and isn't dangerous, and too many situations will seem dangerous that are not. This can fuel your avoidance even more, so you can get caught in a vicious cycle of avoiding situations that are actually safe, never having the opportunity to experience them being safe, and therefore continuing to avoid.

Have you noticed having a fight–flight–freeze reaction in response to trauma triggers— that is, situations that are not actually dangerous but remind you of danger because of your past trauma? What situations or triggers have caused a false alarm of the fight–flight–freeze response for you?

_____

_____

_____

_____

Two 16-year-old friends, James and Mark, were in a severe car accident in which both were injured. The driver, James, blamed himself because he was driving too fast and didn't see the car that hit them drive through the intersection. The accident was not his fault, but he thought that he should have been able to swerve out of the way. His friend, Mark, the passenger, also blamed himself, thinking that he was distracting his friend with his laughing and joking. Both developed PTSD symptoms. After he recovered from his injuries, James refused to drive anymore because he believed driving was dangerous, and his parents went back to driving him everywhere, telling him that the accident proved that he wasn't careful or mature enough to drive yet. Mark was careful after the accident and only drove alone or with his parents in the car for the first few months. Although Mark initially had false alarms of the fight–flight–freeze response when he first got back in the car, because he didn't avoid, he had the chance to learn that most of the time he was safe while driving. Mark's parents encouraged him to drive carefully, of course, but they did encourage him to drive, and after those first few months his PTSD symptoms decreased. James, on the other hand, continued to have nightmares, and his parents were happy to drive him wherever he needed to go, although he went fewer places after that. James continued to have PTSD, whereas Mark recovered within a few months.

This is also a good example of how thinking plays a role in PTSD and recovery. Because of your trauma, you may start to have thoughts about the dangerousness of the world generally or particular places or situations that are based on symptoms of PTSD rather than the actual realistic danger of those situations (because you feel fear, you assume you are in danger and act accordingly). Besides thoughts about dangerousness, many different types of beliefs about ourselves and the world can be affected by traumatic events.

> ▶▶│ Throughout this book we offer you "whiteboard" videos to explain the concepts or demonstrate how to complete the various worksheets. Some people like to learn through reading, while others would rather have a spoken and visual explanation. The videos give you that option. These whiteboard videos are located on the CPT website in the Resources section. To watch a video to review what you just read here about the fight–flight–freeze response and how avoidance can interfere with recovery and keep you "stuck" in PTSD, go to the CPT Whiteboard Video Library (*http://cptforptsd.com/cpt-resources*) and watch the video called

Recovery and Fight or Flight. You may want to bookmark the video library website on your computer so that you can return to it easily to watch additional videos that are suggested throughout this book.

How Thinking Affects Recovery

As you were growing up, you learned about the world and how it works. As that happened, you began to organize the information that was all around you into categories or beliefs. For example, when you were small, you learned that a thing with a back, a seat, and four legs is a chair. In the beginning you may have called a couch a chair or a park bench a chair because they all had a back, a seat, and four legs. Later, as you got older, through experience, you learned to put things into more complex categories. You learned that there are dining room chairs, rocking chairs, recliners, folding chairs, and so forth. This happens for ideas and beliefs about others, the world, and ourselves as well. We start putting things into categories like fun or boring, right or wrong, good or bad, safe or unsafe, fair or unfair. Over time we realize that some things don't fit neatly into simple categories. This happens with the way we think about the traumatic events in our lives, too.

One simple category or way of thinking that many people learn while growing up is that "good things happen to good people, and bad things happen to bad people." This is called the **just-world belief**. It suggests that the world is "just," or fair. You may have learned this belief through your religion, parents, or teachers, or you may have picked it up as a way to make the world seem safer and more predictable. The just-world belief makes sense when you are young. For example, when parents are teaching their children rules, they wouldn't say, "If you do something you're not supposed to, you may or may not get in trouble" or "If you cross the street without holding my hand, you may or not be safe." Therefore, we come to believe that there is a simple cause and effect of our actions and the consequences we experience. However, as we grow up, we realize that the world is more complex than that, and events and circumstances don't always fit our ideas and beliefs about how things "should" happen. Nonetheless, if you have ever had things go badly and thought to yourself "Why me?" then you have experienced the just-world belief. When you ask, "Why me?" you are looking for what you did to deserve an event, and that assumes that outcomes are distributed fairly based on what you did or didn't do. But is that always the case? In fact, "bad" things happen to "good" people, and people sometimes do the "wrong" thing without any consequences. Accidents can happen even when people are trying to be safe. Sometimes we're just in the wrong place at the wrong time. It's also the just-world belief if you ever wondered "Why was *I* spared?" if you experienced a traumatic event in which others were hurt or killed but you survived.

We often hear about people "blaming the victim." This is a way that people use the just-world belief to interpret events in a way that gives them a sense of control. For example, someone who hears of a woman being sexually assaulted at a party might think "What happened to her could never happen to me because I'd be more careful than she was." By assuming that the woman could have prevented it in some way, they blame the victim rather than the person who actually committed the crime. The just-world belief helps them believe that they can keep themselves safe if they do everything "right." We all would like to think that bad events are preventable, but of course they are not always. Contrary to the just-world belief way of thinking, even when we are careful and do what we are supposed to, traumatic events can occur. And sometimes when we aren't as careful as we could be, nothing bad happens.

After a traumatic event, we try to make sense of what happened, either consciously or unconsciously. When an unexpected event occurs that doesn't fit with previous beliefs about the way the world works, there are different ways that we may try to make it fit. One way people try to make the event fit with their previous beliefs is by **changing their memory or interpretation of the event**. Examples include blaming yourself for not preventing the event (or not protecting loved ones), having trouble accepting that the event happened (for example, thinking "If only I hadn't done such-and-such, this wouldn't have happened"), forgetting that it happened or forgetting the most horrifying parts, or questioning your interpretation of what happened (for example, thinking "Maybe it wasn't really abuse"). Changing your interpretation of the event may seem easier than changing your entire set of beliefs about how the world works, how people behave, or your safety. You might say things to yourself like "I should have known that it would happen" or "If I had been more alert, I could have stopped it." Again, these might be ways of holding on to the way you thought the world works, such as trying to believe that bad events are always preventable.

Instead of changing your memory or interpretation of the event, you may need to reexamine how you made sense of what happened. You may come to understand your role in what happened differently once you slow down and look closely at the facts of the event. This is one of the goals in CPT—to help you process and accept what happened in a way that reflects the full reality and context of what happened, and to recognize when old beliefs that aren't realistic or serving you well are getting in the way of your recovery, so that you can change them.

The other way that people make sense of a traumatic event when it doesn't fit with how they thought the world worked is to **go overboard and change their beliefs too much**. If you used to believe that you could control what happens to you but then you experienced a traumatic event in which you didn't have control, you may have begun to believe you have *no* control over what happens to you. If you used to believe that people can be trusted, after a traumatic event, you might begin to believe that *nobody* can be trusted. If you used to believe you were safe in your home or neighborhood but then something traumatic happens there, you may begin to believe that your home or neighborhood is *completely* dangerous. In other words, people start to base all of their expectations about the future on the trauma, not taking into account all of the nontraumatic experiences they had before and since. These extreme changes in thinking might then result in a reluctance to become intimate or develop trust, and increased fear. People often have both of these kinds of shifts in thinking, both changing their interpretation of the event to fit with previous beliefs and changing beliefs to be more extreme.

Those previous examples focused on what happens when people have neutral or positive pretrauma beliefs. However, some people had previous negative experiences in their life and already had negative views of themselves, others, and the world even before the trauma in question. For them, later traumatic events can seem to reinforce or confirm these previously held negative beliefs. For example, prior to having experienced new trauma, you might have believed that you always fail, that others can't be trusted, or that the world is generally unsafe. Then the traumatic event comes along and seems to confirm those beliefs. Or maybe you were told that everything was your fault growing up, so when a bad thing happens, it seems to confirm that, once again, you are at fault. In this case, it may be necessary to figure out what your actual degree of safety, control, or ability to trust yourself or others is within your current circumstances.

Larissa was adopted at a young age because her parents had problems with drug use. Because she had this experience, she already had thoughts like "I'm not important" and "I'm not worth sticking around for" when thinking about why her parents used drugs and could not take care of her. When Larissa was in high school, her best friend died by suicide. In making sense of why her friend died by suicide, Larissa felt sad and guilty and thought "I should have done more to help her," but she also felt angry at her friend and had thoughts like "She didn't even care how I would be affected" and "I wasn't worth staying alive for." In a way, Larissa's interpretation of the trauma was influenced by her thoughts about her earlier experiences. She tended to assume that bad things that happened to her occurred because of something about her, such as that she wasn't "good" enough, important enough, or lovable enough. These ways of thinking about trauma are all based on the just-world belief because they assume that there is a logical or fair reason why things happen or that bad things happen in response to people being bad or unworthy.

In reality, Larissa's friend's suicide wasn't about Larissa at all. In fact, her friend had been suffering from depression for a long time and couldn't or didn't get the help that she needed. And, of course, Larissa's parents didn't use drugs because Larissa wasn't important; it was that they had an addiction. Because of her experiences, Larissa also developed more negative beliefs about herself, others, and the world generally. She generally thought about herself, "I'm not lovable." With regard to others, she thought "Other people will always leave you." These thoughts weren't based on all of her experiences, but based on her most negative, traumatic experiences. As Larissa worked through her traumas, she began to examine her assumptions about why the events actually occurred and what they really meant about her and others.

Overall, a key goal of CPT is to help you identify and accept the reality of your traumatic experience, including why it really happened and what it means that it happened, based on the facts of the situation. This involves developing balanced and realistic beliefs about the event, yourself, and others. An additional goal is to allow yourself to feel the emotions resulting from the reality of the event so that you can move toward recovery. The next section discusses different kinds of emotions and how you'll address them in this process.

▶▶ To watch a video to review what you just read here about how the way we think affects recovery, go to the CPT Whiteboard Video Library (*http://cptforptsd.com/ cpt-resources*) and watch the video called *Cognitive Theory*.

Types of Emotions

There are two kinds of emotions that follow traumatic events. The first type includes the feelings that follow naturally from an event and would be universal, with no thought required: fear when in real danger, anger when being intentionally harmed, joy or happiness with positive events, or sadness with losses. These **natural emotions** have a natural course. They won't continue at the same intensity forever. After you allow yourself to experience them, they dissipate. It's important for your recovery to feel these emotions that you may not have allowed yourself to experience about the event and let them run their course.

The second type of emotions, which we call **manufactured emotions**, result not directly from the event but from your interpretations of the event. They are *not* called "manufactured" because you are "making them up" but because the emotion is manufactured (or created) by a specific thought, like a little factory in your mind. For example, if the traumatic event was that your apartment building was on fire, you may have experienced terror when you realized you were in danger and sadness when you remember what happened. Those would be natural emotions. But if you now have thoughts such as "I should have rescued other people" or "I must be a failure because I can't get over it," you may be feeling guilt or anger with yourself. These emotions may not be based on the facts of the event (that your home was on fire) but on your interpretations (that you didn't do enough to help others or that you should be "over it" by now). The more you continue to think about the event in these ways the more manufactured feelings you are going to have. The bright side is that if your beliefs and interpretations change, so will your feelings.

Think of your emotions as a fire in a fireplace. The fire has energy and heat to it, just like your emotions, but it will burn out if it's not continually fed. In other words, if you let yourself feel the natural emotions (such as sadness that it happened or anger at a perpetrator), those emotions will eventually fade over time. However, self-blame or guilty thoughts are like logs that can continue to feed the emotional fire indefinitely. Take away the fuel of your thoughts and the fire burns out quickly. For you to recover from your traumatic event(s), it's important to let yourself feel your natural emotions and examine your thoughts underlying the manufactured feelings. You'll do this by getting the full picture of what happened and by taking a close look at what you're saying to yourself now about the event and your role in it, and what it means about you, others, and your future.

Matt was robbed at gunpoint. He was blindsided and feared for his life. The perpetrators began hitting him when he didn't reach for his wallet fast enough. Later he had thoughts like "If I had just given them my wallet faster, they wouldn't have hurt me" and "I should have fought back. I acted like a coward." He felt ashamed whenever he remembered the traumatic event. The shame is an example of a manufactured emotion. As Matt began to work through these thoughts, he realized some important things about the event. First, when it happened, he had an automatic freeze response, so he couldn't reach for his wallet right away. Second, fighting back may have resulted in his getting shot, or injured worse, because there were multiple perpetrators and at least one gun. Matt's thoughts were based less on the full reality of what happened and more on his just-world belief that if something bad happened to him, he must have done something wrong to deserve it. His new thoughts, based on the full context of the event, were "I did the best I could in a dangerous situation where I was surprised and terrified" and "It makes sense that I didn't fight back because I was outnumbered." When he began to think this way, he noticed that he no longer felt ashamed (the manufactured emotion) when he remembered what happened.

▶▶| To watch a video to review what you just read here about emotions, go to the CPT Whiteboard Video Library (*http://cptforptsd.com/cpt-resources*) and watch the video called *Types of Emotions*.

How CPT Works: Examining Stuck Points

Thoughts like those Matt first had are part of what can keep you "stuck" in PTSD, by fueling those manufactured emotions like guilt and shame. Therefore, we call them **stuck points**. Stuck points are thoughts or beliefs, not facts, that lead to strong negative emotions and keep you stuck in PTSD.

One goal of CPT is to help you recognize and modify your stuck points, those things you are saying to yourself about the traumatic event(s) that keep you from moving forward. Most of your thoughts are probably helpful to you. However, there may be some ways of thinking about the trauma that have been less helpful to you or aren't realistic. Those are the kinds of thoughts you'll examine in this book. Your thoughts and interpretations about the event may have become so automatic that you aren't even aware that you have them. Even though you may not be aware of what you are saying to yourself, your beliefs and self-statements affect your mood and your behavior.

For example, as you started to read this book, you probably had questions or thoughts about whether this would work for you. What thoughts did you have about this approach, and what emotions did you feel?

_____

_____

_____

_____

You may have noticed some thoughts like "This will never work," "I'm too messed up for this to help," "Writing my thoughts down about the event will make the event real," or "I'll never get the hang of it." These are examples of stuck points that are not directly related to the traumatic event, but that happen in the here-and-now and can interfere with your recovery. If you act on these thoughts, you may end up not giving this book or other treatment a fair shot. This can keep you stuck. You may also notice thoughts like "I can't handle memories of the trauma." Stuck points like this may lead you to avoid doing the work in this book. We cannot emphasize enough how important it is that you not avoid. This will be your biggest (and probably scariest) hurdle. You can't feel your feelings or examine your thoughts if you avoid practicing the skills that you're learning.

In the next chapter, you'll identify what your specific stuck points are and how they influence what you feel. You'll learn ways to examine and change what you are saying to yourself and what you believe about yourself and the event. Some of your beliefs about the event will be more balanced or realistic than others. You'll focus on the stuck points—the beliefs that are interfering with your recovery or keeping you stuck with your PTSD. You'll identify and write down your stuck points in a log in this book so that when you work on exploring your beliefs in later chapters, you'll have this list to draw on.

Focusing on Your Index Event

In Chapter 2 you identified your index event—the traumatic event that you consider to be the worst, or the one that is haunting you the most, causing most of your PTSD symptoms, or most at the root of your PTSD symptoms. You used this index event to fill out the Base-line PTSD Checklist on pages 14–15, and this event will be the one that you use to complete the activities throughout this book, at least to begin with.

Why focus on the worst traumatic event? If you work on your most distressing trau-matic event, you are likely to get the most benefit from this process. If you start with a less traumatic event, at the end of your work, you may feel better about that secondary event but will likely still have to go back to work on the one that causes the most PTSD symp-toms. Many people who have PTSD have had more than one traumatic event, and you can absolutely address more than one traumatic event in this process. You should start with the worst event, however, because if you tackle that one, you can begin to apply what you have learned to the other traumatic events, about which you may have similar thoughts and emo-tions. Often when you start working on the worst traumatic event first, you'll see benefits in how you think about the others as well.

As we noted in Chapter 2, some people know right away which event is bothering them the most. If that wasn't the case for you, we gave you a timeline to chronicle all of your traumatic experiences as well as some questions to help you decide which one to focus on. Chances are you've been living with the event, having flashbacks or nightmares and strong emotions when reminded of it, trying to push it away or avoid it whenever you can. In fact, you have been coping with it, but not in the way that would help you recover. If you haven't identified an index event yet, go back to page 11 now to select an event before moving on to the next exercise. Again, however, don't delay getting started with the work out of inde-cision about which event to start with. Choose the one you think you'll benefit most from addressing and then continue with the next step in this book.

Of course, just thinking about the sad and scary things that have happened to you can bring up a lot of emotions. But stick with it. Now is no time to turn back, before you've even had a chance to benefit from your efforts so far. A major purpose of CPT is to help you live with and accept that this event happened but reduce the strong emotions that get in the way of you living your life.

PRACTICE ASSIGNMENT

The first assignment will help you start identifying how you think about your worst traumatic event. The assignment (which you will find on pages 47–48 and online at *www.guilford.com/resick2-forms*) is called the Impact Statement because you'll identify how the event has impacted your thinking. You are not going to be asked to write the details of what happened. Instead, you'll focus on your current thoughts about the event so that you know what to focus on in the rest of this process. This is not like a class assignment in school, so don't worry about things like spelling or grammar. The important thing is to just do it. It has also been found that writing your Impact Statement by hand is better than typing it. Writing it by hand will slow you down to help you think about it in more depth. Keyboarding it into a computer adds distance (which could function as avoidance), and you can get caught up in grammar and spell-checking.

For this assignment to be most helpful, we strongly suggest you start as soon as possible so you won't be tempted to put it off or avoid. Can you start it right now? If so, do so. Most of the clients we work with are anxious about doing this assignment. So, almost certainly there will be an urge to avoid. But now is an important time to overcome that urge for the purpose of getting better. Avoiding right now would be like sitting on a fence, somewhere between fully avoiding and doing the work completely. Sitting on a fence is not a comfortable place to be! You've come this far, so go all in, like jumping into a pool or ripping off a bandage.

You don't have to write your Impact Statement all in one sitting. You can keep adding to it over a number of days as you think about it. But don't spend too long trying to "perfect" your statement. The important part is to get your thoughts down on paper so you can see why you think that the event happened and what the outcomes have been in your thinking and your life. The sooner you start, the more likely that you will not avoid and will be able to keep moving toward recovery. So, turn to the Impact Statement and start the assignment as soon as possible—now, if you can. After you get your responses down, you can move on to Chapter 5.

 TROUBLESHOOTING

What if I can't pick a worst event? They were all similar.

Even though they seem similar or equally distressing, try to pick a single event to focus on first. If you try to focus on a whole group of traumatic events, your thoughts will be more vague. If you focus on a single event, you'll be able to identify the specific thoughts you have about why that exact event happened and identify specific stuck points to work on. In a series of events, like, for example, multiple instances of domestic violence by an abusive romantic partner, the most shocking and PTSD-producing event might have been the very first one. However, if the perpetrator apologized and said it would never happen again, and it didn't happen again for a long time, that might not be the worst incident. The one that causes the most PTSD symptoms might be one that stands out because the perpetrator broke that promise, there was forced sexual contact, you were badly injured and/or thought you were going to die, or the perpetrator started abusing the children, too.

Impact Statement

Please write at least one page on *why* you think your worst traumatic event occurred. You are *not* being asked to write specifics about the traumatic event. Write about what you have been thinking about the *cause* of the worst event.

Here are some questions that might be helpful to consider as you write about the cause of the event:

- Who have you been thinking is to blame for this event?
- Have you been thinking of things you should have done differently? If so, what?
- Have you been thinking of things other people should have done differently? If so, what?
- Have you been thinking the event could have been prevented? If so, how?
- Why do you think this event happened to you (versus to someone else)?
- What does it mean about you that this event happened?
- If the event happened to someone else, why do you think it happened to them (versus to another person)?

Also, consider the *effects* this traumatic event has had on your beliefs about yourself, others, and the world in the following areas: safety, trust, power/control, esteem, and intimacy. You can write your responses to the questions about why the event happened and the effects of the trauma in the space below.

_____

_____

_____

_____

_____

_____

_____

_____

_____

_____

_____

_____

_____

(continued)

Think back and see if one event pops into your mind first and ask yourself why. That may be the key. Also, if there is one event that you work harder to push away, or if there is one that you feel the most guilt or shame about, that could be the index event, the place to start. If a couple of events really seem equal to you, then you could start with the earliest one. But remember, if you start with an "easier" one, it won't help you recover from the worst event, whereas if you start with the worst one, the work you do on that event is likely to extend to the "easier" events, too. Keep in mind that if there are different stuck points from other traumatic events, you can work with them later in the process. Your stuck points are likely to be similar with later traumatic events. As noted earlier, you'll have the opportunity to work on multiple events.

What if I don't want to stop avoiding?

It's understandable to want to avoid. No one likes to think about the worst things that have happened to them or feel emotions like fear, sadness, and anger. However, you may want to remind yourself that while avoidance may work in the short run, in the long run it keeps the PTSD stuck. Unfortunately, research suggests that people don't spontaneously recover from PTSD once they have it, and we have seen people in therapy who had PTSD since World War II. If you don't think about it intentionally, you are likely to continue to have trauma memories pop up and interfere with your life. Perhaps it's time to work on the trauma so that you can have control over the memories instead of their having control over you. Refer back to your goals in the previous section and remind yourself why you wanted to give this a try. What if not avoiding for a few weeks or months meant that you could substantially reduce your PTSD symptoms and get on track toward your goals? Would it be worth it?

I am having trouble starting my Impact Statement. How do I write it without writing about the traumatic event?

Remember that you are writing about *what you have been saying to yourself* about the causes and consequences of the traumatic event, not the details of what happened. Naturally you will think about the event while you think about the causes of the event, and it is not dangerous to think about the event, but the purpose of the Impact Statement is to identify your thoughts about the event, so you can just use a short term for it (for example, *the shooting, being beaten, the hurricane, the rape, the car accident, my friend being killed in front of me*). Don't use a vague term like *the event* or *that day,* because naming it specifically will help you accept it better. Remember that there are no wrong answers. This is an activity designed to help you begin to identify your thoughts.

What if I don't know what to say about why it happened?

Chances are you have been saying something to yourself about why it happened, even if it happened when you were very young or you don't know the actual reason why it happened. The activities in this book will help you sort out whether your thought is accurate, but for now, just write down why you think it happened when you think about it. This might include what you have been telling yourself about why it happened, or what others have told you about why it happened that you believe, like "I was abused because I was bad" or "It happened because I didn't listen" or "I shouldn't have trusted him." If you haven't been letting yourself think about the trauma, this is an opportunity to reflect on what you think about the cause of the trauma. Even if you're saying to yourself "I don't know what I did to deserve the abuse," that suggests you might have a belief like "I must have done something to deserve the abuse." Use the additional questions at the top of the Impact Statement assignment on page 47 to help you get started. In the next chapter, we ask some additional questions that may help you uncover your thoughts about why it happened.

What if I don't know what happened? Can I use this book if I don't completely remember it?

Yes, it's possible to use the skills in this book and recover from PTSD without remembering all or even any of the details of the event. If you were drugged, knocked unconscious, or drunk, for example, you may never get the memory back because it wouldn't have been stored in long-term memory. If you don't remember because you dissociate when you think about it, you may remember more as you stop avoiding. Either way, the important part is that you know that the event did happen and you have thoughts and emotions about it. That is what you will focus on in this process.

What if I don't have any stuck points?

It's very rare for someone who has PTSD not to have any stuck points. However, if you have not been allowing yourself to feel your natural emotions or have been avoiding your memories of the traumatic events, you may be unaware of what your thoughts are. It's also possible that you are considering your stuck points to be facts right now. If you have guilt, shame, or anger at yourself or at someone who did not directly cause the event, you probably do have stuck points. Writing the Impact Statement should help you identify your stuck points. The next chapter also walks you through how to identify stuck points.

   Important! *Start this as soon as possible, right now if you can.* Starting is often the hardest part, but the anxiety anticipating the activity may be worse than actually doing it. Once you get going, you may surprise yourself that you are able to do it. Taking this step will allow you to move toward recovery. If you need to, look back at the goals you set to remind yourself of why you are doing this. Don't quit now! If you keep going, you could be feeling better within a few weeks.

*   *   *

   Why fill out the PTSD Checklist each week? Tracking your symptoms allows you to see how your symptoms are improving as you progress through the book. If your symptoms are not improving by Chapter 8, you can assess whether avoidance or anything else has gotten in the way. It will also help you decide when you have benefited enough and are ready to graduate. Remember to track your progress using the Graph for Tracking Your Weekly Scores found on page 24.

PTSD Checklist

Complete the PTSD Checklist to track your symptoms as you complete this book. Be sure to complete this measure on the same index event each time. When the instructions and questions refer to a "stressful experience," remember that that is your index event—the worst event that you are working on first.

Write in here the trauma that you are working on first: _____

Complete this PTSD Checklist with reference to that event.

Instructions: Below is a list of problems that people sometimes have in response to a very stressful experience. Please read each problem carefully, and then circle one of the numbers to the right to indicate how much you have been bothered by that problem *in the past week.*

In the past week, how much were you bothered by:	Not at all	A little bit	Mod- erately	Quite a bit	Extremely
1. Repeated, disturbing, and unwanted memories of the stressful experience?	0	1	2	3	4
2. Repeated, disturbing dreams of the stressful experience?	0	1	2	3	4
3. Suddenly feeling or acting as if the stressful experience were actually happening again (*as if you were actually back there reliving it*)?	0	1	2	3	4
4. Feeling very upset when something reminded you of the stressful experience?	0	1	2	3	4
5. Having strong physical reactions when something reminded you of the stressful experience (*for example, heart pounding, trouble breathing, sweating*)?	0	1	2	3	4
6. Avoiding memories, thoughts, or feelings related to the stressful experience?	0	1	2	3	4
7. Avoiding external reminders of the stressful experience (*for example, people, places, conversations, activities, objects, or situations*)?	0	1	2	3	4
8. Trouble remembering important parts of the stressful experience (not due to head injury or substances)?	0	1	2	3	4
9. Having strong negative beliefs about yourself, other people, or the world (*for example, having thoughts such as I am bad, There is something seriously wrong with me, No one can be trusted, or The world is completely dangerous*)?	0	1	2	3	4
10. Blaming yourself or someone else (who didn't intend the outcome) for the stressful experience or what happened after it?	0	1	2	3	4
11. Having strong negative feelings, such as fear, horror, anger, guilt, or shame?	0	1	2	3	4
12. Loss of interest in activities that you used to enjoy?	0	1	2	3	4
13. Feeling distant or cut off from other people?	0	1	2	3	4
14. Trouble experiencing positive feelings (*for example, being unable to feel happiness or have loving feelings for people close to you*)?	0	1	2	3	4
15. Irritable behavior, angry outbursts, or acting aggressively?	0	1	2	3	4
16. Taking too many risks or doing things that could cause you harm?	0	1	2	3	4
17. Being "super alert" or watchful or on guard?	0	1	2	3	4
18. Feeling jumpy or easily startled?	0	1	2	3	4
19. Having difficulty concentrating?	0	1	2	3	4
20. Trouble falling or staying asleep?	0	1	2	3	4

Add up the total and write it here: _____

From *PTSD Checklist for DSM-5 (PCL-5)* by Weathers, Litz, Keane, Palmieri, Marx, and Schnurr (2013). Available from the National Center for PTSD at *www.ptsd.va.gov*; in the public domain. Reprinted in *Getting Unstuck from PTSD* (Guilford Press, 2023). Purchasers of this book can photocopy and/or download additional copies of this worksheet at *www.guilford.com/resick2-forms* for personal use or use with clients; see copyright page for details.

5

Processing the Meaning of Your Trauma and Building a Stuck Point Log

Congratulations on writing your Impact Statement! How was it for you to complete this activity? Give yourself a lot of credit for completing this assignment; doing so means you did not avoid facing the difficult memories and emotions that may have come along with it. Because you have done the work to explore your thoughts related to the trauma, you have taken a big step toward identifying where you may have gotten stuck in your recovery. The next step is to build a list of your stuck points—your Stuck Point Log—which will guide the rest of your work. Once you identify your personal stuck points, you can use the skills in the chapters that follow to address them one by one and process the trauma.

If you have not yet completed your Impact Statement (pages 47–48), go back and do that now before moving on to this chapter. The Impact Statement and Stuck Point Log are crucial to CPT, so be sure to stay focused and get these done so that you can continue on the road to recovery.

> Lina felt overwhelmed while looking at the Impact Statement prompt. She had been avoiding thinking about her trauma for decades, and she didn't know where to begin when thinking about "why" it happened. Lina became a refugee when she was forced to flee her home country, but her sister and brother-in-law were not able to get out and were ultimately killed in the conflict. At first, she put her book away and figured she would come back to it the next day. But the next day, she felt an even greater urge to avoid thinking about the trauma and cleaned her apartment instead. A couple of days later, Lina had a panic attack at the grocery store and decided she needed to work through her trauma so that she didn't feel so overwhelmed in her daily life. Lina wasn't sure what to write, but she followed the suggestions in the book not to worry about writing a "perfect" response and just got her thoughts down on paper. She used the questions at the top of the Impact Statement to help get her thinking about whether she felt to blame or had any "should haves." She realized that although she typically avoided thinking about

it, she had thoughts like "I shouldn't have left them behind" and "If I had stayed behind to help them, they would still be alive." Having completed the Impact Statement, Lina was well on her way to identifying the stuck points that she needed to examine to address her PTSD.

Remember that a stuck point is a thought or belief that may not be one hundred percent fact but that leads to negative emotions and gets in the way of recovery. In this chapter, you'll use your Impact Statement and some of the guides and questions provided to figure out what you have been telling yourself about the trauma that might be a stuck point. Then you'll write them down on your Stuck Point Log (a blank form is provided on page 56, or you can download and print the Stuck Point Log from *www.guilford.com/resick2-forms*). It's very likely that some of your thoughts about the trauma are accurate and helpful and therefore not stuck points. What you want to identify now are the thoughts that are less helpful and are getting in the way of your recovery—those are your stuck points. If in doubt about whether something is a stuck point, write it down anyway. You can explore it more later. If you are unsure about your stuck points, that's OK. Just keep going. The book will guide you. The important thing is to keep at it and not give up.

There are two main kinds of stuck points to look for. The first are the thoughts that may be related to the first part of your Impact Statement: thoughts about *why the trauma happened, what the cause of the trauma was, who is to blame,* and *whether it could have been prevented.*

The other kind of stuck point may be related to the second part of your Impact Statement: *how you have been thinking about yourself, others, and the world as a result of your traumatic experience.* These are extreme thoughts about the present and the future.

Stuck Points about the Traumatic Event

The first category of stuck points is typically about the past, such as why the trauma happened, whether it could have been prevented, and so on. These may include the following:

- **Shoulda–coulda–wouldas**
  - For example, "I should have known my daughter was using drugs again" or "I could have stopped it."
- **If onlys**
  - For example, "If only I had seen the red flags, I never would have been assaulted" or "If only I had been there, I could have stopped my friend from being killed."
- **Self-blame** for something you did not actually want to happen
  - For example, "It's my fault my friend died" or "I am to blame for my husband's suicide."
- **Blaming people or factors** that were not the main cause
  - For example, "It's my dad's fault that my mother abused us because he left her" or "Our commander was to blame for ordering us to drive down that road in Iraq."

- **Just-world beliefs** (see Chapter 4) that assume there is fairness in who experiences a trauma
  - For example, "I must have done something to deserve it" or "It shouldn't have happened to him because he had a family."

Looking over your Impact Statement, or thinking about your index trauma now, what stuck points like these might you have? Where have you been placing the blame for the event? What *shoulda–coulda–wouldas* and *if onlys* have been going through your mind?

Stuck points should be full sentences, not questions or single words or phrases. Make sure that each one is a single thought, not multiple ideas contained in a single sentence. Also, stuck points by definition are not facts. So, while it may be a fact that you feel emotions or engage in certain behaviors, try to focus on what the thought is behind your thoughts and emotions. Refer to the box on the facing page for tips and examples on how to word your stuck points. Then add your thoughts to your Stuck Point Log (see page 56).

Stuck Points Resulting from the Trauma

The other kind of stuck point has more to do with your general beliefs, which may have become more negative since the trauma. You may have written about these in the second part of your Impact Statement when you wrote about the effects of the trauma on your beliefs about safety, trust, power/control, esteem, and intimacy. These may include the following:

- **Predictions about the future**, assuming what "will" happen
  - For example, "If I trust someone, I will be hurt" or "If I go out at night, I will be assaulted."
- **Generalizations** with words like *always, all, everyone, never, no one,* and the like
  - For example, "No one can be trusted," "The world is completely dangerous," or "I always fail."

Looking over your Impact Statement, or thinking about it now, what stuck points like these do you have? What assumptions have you been making about the future? What generalizations have you made about yourself, others, and the world?

On page 57 is an example from Pablo, who wrote his Impact Statement and then used that to build his Stuck Point Log.

Once you have had a chance to go through your Impact Statement and identify your stuck points, you may also refer to the checklist on pages 55–56 to see if there are any other stuck points you may have. If any of these common stuck points ring true for you, add them to your Stuck Point Log as well. Also refer to the Resources at the end of the book for common stuck points that people with different types of traumatic experiences often have.

Tips for Wording Your Stuck Points

Tip	Less helpful wording	More helpful wording
Write your stuck point as a complete statement.	*Trust*	*I shouldn't have trusted him.*
Rephrase questions into statements. Sometimes it helps to ask yourself what your answer is to your question.	*Why did I go to his house?*	*I shouldn't have gone to his house.*
Try to have each stuck point contain only one main idea. Split up your thought into multiple stuck points if needed.	*It happened because I was stupid, weak, and drunk.*	*It happened because I was stupid.* *It happened because I was weak.* *It happened because I was drunk.*
Notice if you are saying something tentative, such as what "may" happen, if what you *really* think is more definite.	*If I trust someone, I **may** be hurt again.* (Possibly true—anything "may" happen.)	*If I trust someone, I **will** be hurt again.*
Look for the thoughts behind your behaviors and emotions.	*I rarely go out of the house.* *When I go out, I feel afraid.* (It may be true that you engage in that behavior or feel that emotion, but what are you saying to yourself that leads to that emotion or behavior?)	*If I go out, I will be attacked.*

Stuck Point Log

_____

_____

_____

_____

_____

_____

_____

_____

_____

_____

_____

_____

_____

_____

_____

_____

_____

_____

_____

_____

_____

_____

Example Impact Statement

The physical abuse by my grandmother happened because my mother left me with her. My mother must have known my grandmother would abuse me, but she left me there anyway. Maybe she didn't care. The worst time my grandmother abused me, it happened because I didn't come right home from school like she told me to do. She said she needed to teach me to behave. I should have just come home. If I had, it might not have happened. Because of the way I grew up, I have never felt good enough. I feel unlikable and incompetent. Also, if your own family can abuse or abandon you, then how can I think anyone will ever really care for me? Every time I think about opening up to someone, I get afraid and think they will hurt me, too.

Example Stuck Point Log

It's my mother's fault I was abused.

My mother must have known I would be abused.

I wasn't worth taking care of.

I should have come right home from school.

I deserved the abuse.

If only I had behaved, I would not have been abused.

I am not good enough.

I am unlikable.

I am incompetent.

No one will ever really care for me.

If I open up to someone, they will hurt me.

Common Stuck Points about the Traumatic Event

❏ It's my fault the event happened.

❏ The event happened because of something about me.

❏ I must have done something to deserve the event.

❏ It happened because I did/didn't _____.

❑ The event happened as punishment (from God, karma, etc.).

❑ Bad things happen because you've done something wrong.

❑ Things are supposed to be fair.

❑ Things like this aren't supposed to happen to _____ (good/innocent people, kids, etc.).

❑ I could have prevented it.

❑ I should/could have stopped it.

The more specific you can make the stuck point the better. So, if you think "The event happened because of something about me," do you have ideas about specifically what it is about you? If so, write that down on your Stuck Point Log. For example, some people think "It happened because I was weak," "It happened because I had bad judgment," "It happened because I wasn't worth protecting," or "It happened because I attract bad events/people."

It's important to remember that we are writing these thoughts down because they are not necessarily true. Yet these are the thoughts that may circle around your head and keep you stuck in PTSD. By writing them down on your Stuck Point Log, you are taking a big step toward recovery. You'll have the chance to consider each of them more carefully as you make your way through the rest of the book. So keep up the good work and keep going!

Common Stuck Points Resulting from the Trauma

Safety

❑ The world is completely dangerous.

❑ If I'm not on guard, something terrible will happen.

❑ I can't keep myself safe.

❑ Crowds are dangerous.

Trust

❑ No one is trustworthy.

❑ If I trust someone, they will hurt me.

❑ I can't trust my judgment.

Power/Control

❑ If I'm not in control at all times, something terrible will happen.

❑ I'm powerless to prevent bad things from happening to me.

❑ Other people will try to control me if I let them.

Esteem

❑ I am damaged.

❑ I am broken.

❑ I should be over this by now.

❑ I will never get any better.

❑ I am unlovable.

❑ No one cares about me.

❑ No one can understand me.

❑ Other people are basically selfish and uncaring.

❑ If someone is nice, they always have ulterior motives.

Intimacy

❑ If I let my guard down with someone, they will hurt me.

❑ If I let myself feel my emotions, I will lose control.

❑ I can't cope without _____ (alcohol, drugs, comfort food, etc.).

❑ Sex is dangerous.

Again, if any of these ring true for you, add them to your Stuck Point Log. If you have completed this step, you now have a list of thoughts that you can address to move toward trauma recovery. Great work! You are now ready to begin taking a closer look at these thoughts and how they affect how you feel. Bookmark your Stuck Point Log, because you'll continue to refer back to it in each chapter and may add to it later.

> ▶▶ To watch a video to review what you have read here about stuck points, go to the CPT Whiteboard Video Library (*http://cptforptsd.com/cpt-resources*) and watch the videos called *What Are Stuck Points?* and *How Do I Identify Stuck Points?*

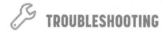 **TROUBLESHOOTING**

I don't understand what to put on the Stuck Point Log.

You are just learning what stuck points are, so don't worry if you don't totally understand the concept yet. If you feel confused, you can always reread the chapter or watch the videos. However, you'll continue to learn more about stuck points and what to do with them in the chapters ahead, so once you have some stuck points down on your log you can proceed to the next chapter. If you aren't sure what to put on your log, reread the list of common stuck points on the previous pages and also refer to the Resources, where there are examples of stuck points for different kinds of traumatic events. You can start by checking off any of the statements that you believe and adding them to your Stuck Point Log. Then go back and look at your Impact Statement. What did you say was the cause of the event? Are there any other thoughts that might be worth adding to your log so that you can examine them later?

How many stuck points should I have? Do I have too many? Do I have too few?

There is no right or wrong number of stuck points to have on your log. When you are first building your Stuck Point Log, a reasonable number to shoot for is ten to twenty statements. However, some people have only a handful of stuck points and some people have many more (seventy-five to eighty). Do nonetheless make sure that you didn't skip over identifying stuck points about why the trauma happened. Try to come up with at least a few stuck points about why the trauma happened, and a few about what it means about yourself, others, the world, or your future. As you continue in the book, you may identify more stuck points, and you can always go back and add them to your log. Even if they sound similar to another one you wrote down, write down any stuck points that come to mind. Sometimes a slight change in wording (for example, writing both "It's my fault because I went out that night" and "I should have stayed home that night") can help you later when you are examining the thought.

Looking over this list of stuck points, I'm starting to feel overwhelmed.

It's common to feel overwhelmed while looking at your list of stuck points. However, consider it this way: You now have a list of the thoughts that have gotten in the way of your recovery. Instead of just whirling around in your head, now the thoughts are on paper, where you can see them and take control over them. You now have a road map for where you need to go to get unstuck from your PTSD. You've completed the first step of identifying your stuck points. The rest of this book will help you work through them one by one.

I don't believe my thoughts are wrong. They are true.

At this point in the process, you are not evaluating whether your thoughts are true. Just write down any beliefs or thoughts you have about the most distressing traumatic event (your index event). You'll have a chance to evaluate them later. It's possible that some are true. You'll evaluate the evidence and decide for yourself later in the process. If they are, you'll get help figuring out what to do to move forward.

*   *   *

Remember that tracking your symptoms each week is a helpful way to monitor your progress. Continue tracking your scores using the Graph for Tracking Your Weekly Scores on page 24. You may not be feeling better yet because you have only just gotten started, but you may be able to notice if you are at least decreasing your avoidance (items 6 and 7 on the PTSD Checklist). If you have an increase in your intrusive symptoms, it's probably because you are reducing your avoidance. This is progress!

(PTSD Checklist)

Complete the PTSD Checklist to track your symptoms as you complete this book. Be sure to complete this measure on the same index event each time. When the instructions and questions refer to a "stressful experience," remember that that is your index event—the worst event that you are working on first.

Write in here the trauma that you are working on first: _____

Complete this PTSD Checklist with reference to that event.

Instructions: Below is a list of problems that people sometimes have in response to a very stressful experience. Please read each problem carefully, and then circle one of the numbers to the right to indicate how much you have been bothered by that problem *in the past week*.

In the past week, how much were you bothered by:	Not at all	A little bit	Mod- erately	Quite a bit	Extremely
1. Repeated, disturbing, and unwanted memories of the stressful experience?	0	1	2	3	4
2. Repeated, disturbing dreams of the stressful experience?	0	1	2	3	4
3. Suddenly feeling or acting as if the stressful experience were actually happening again (*as if you were actually back there reliving it*)?	0	1	2	3	4
4. Feeling very upset when something reminded you of the stressful experience?	0	1	2	3	4
5. Having strong physical reactions when something reminded you of the stressful experience (*for example, heart pounding, trouble breathing, sweating*)?	0	1	2	3	4
6. Avoiding memories, thoughts, or feelings related to the stressful experience?	0	1	2	3	4
7. Avoiding external reminders of the stressful experience (*for example, people, places, conversations, activities, objects, or situations*)?	0	1	2	3	4
8. Trouble remembering important parts of the stressful experience (not due to head injury or substances)?	0	1	2	3	4
9. Having strong negative beliefs about yourself, other people, or the world (*for example, having thoughts such as I am bad, There is something seriously wrong with me, No one can be trusted, or The world is completely dangerous*)?	0	1	2	3	4
10. Blaming yourself or someone else (who didn't intend the outcome) for the stressful experience or what happened after it?	0	1	2	3	4
11. Having strong negative feelings, such as fear, horror, anger, guilt, or shame?	0	1	2	3	4
12. Loss of interest in activities that you used to enjoy?	0	1	2	3	4
13. Feeling distant or cut off from other people?	0	1	2	3	4
14. Trouble experiencing positive feelings (*for example, being unable to feel happiness or have loving feelings for people close to you*)?	0	1	2	3	4
15. Irritable behavior, angry outbursts, or acting aggressively?	0	1	2	3	4
16. Taking too many risks or doing things that could cause you harm?	0	1	2	3	4
17. Being "super alert" or watchful or on guard?	0	1	2	3	4
18. Feeling jumpy or easily startled?	0	1	2	3	4
19. Having difficulty concentrating?	0	1	2	3	4
20. Trouble falling or staying asleep?	0	1	2	3	4

Add up the total and write it here: _____

From *PTSD Checklist for DSM-5 (PCL-5)* by Weathers, Litz, Keane, Palmieri, Marx, and Schnurr (2013). Available from the National Center for PTSD at *www.ptsd.va.gov*; in the public domain. Reprinted in *Getting Unstuck from PTSD* (Guilford Press, 2023). Purchasers of this book can photocopy and/or download additional copies of this worksheet at *www.guilford.com/resick2-forms* for personal use or use with clients; see copyright page for details.

6

Identifying Thoughts and Feelings

In Chapter 5 you processed your Impact Statement and built your Stuck Point Log. This is great progress! You have now identified the thoughts to work on to recover from PTSD. Next you'll start to look at how your stuck points and other thoughts that run through your mind may lead you to feel strong negative emotions, like guilt, shame, anger, and fear.

If you have not yet built your Stuck Point Log, go back to Chapter 5 and do that before moving on to this chapter. The Stuck Point Log is very important for the remainder of your work.

Identifying Emotions

There are many kinds of emotions that can be experienced to varying degrees. We have many words to describe what kinds of feelings we are experiencing and how much. Some people are very good at identifying and naming their emotions, and some people are less clear on what emotions they are feeling. Like other skills, it may take practice to be able to recognize and name your emotions and then notice how they may be linked to events and thoughts. This may be especially true if you have avoided emotions.

Although many people with PTSD avoid emotions, feeling numb may not be the best approach because then you don't get to experience positive emotions. We can't block out negative emotions without also restricting our more positive emotions, and that means not feeling as much happiness, joy, and contentment as you could be feeling. This may contribute to feeling detached from others. The goal is to identify where your emotions are coming from and then decide what to do with them to get unstuck from PTSD. If you are feeling a natural emotion—a universal response to the situation, like sadness when there is a loss—then the goal is to feel those emotions until they decrease. If your emotions are based on your thoughts, such as feeling guilty when you think "The event was my fault," then the goal will be to take a closer look at the thought behind the emotion—those thoughts will be the focus of the worksheets that are introduced throughout the rest of this book. The first step, however, is to be able to recognize your emotions and where they are coming from.

The Identifying Emotions diagram on the facing page shows some different emotions, each ranging in intensity from no emotion to extremes of the emotion. There are many

Identifying Emotions

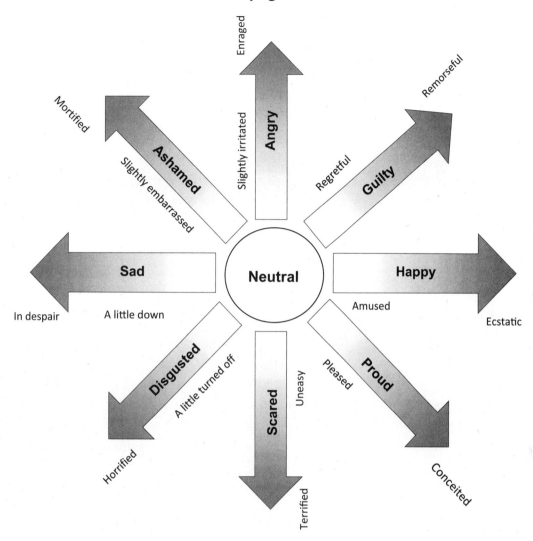

words that could be added along the arms of each emotion. Over time you'll notice that emotions are not just on or off, nothing or extreme. They come in varying intensities depending on the situation or what you are saying to yourself about the situation.

If you have trouble identifying your emotions, notice the physical responses in your body. When you are angry, your heart may race and your muscles bunch up. Are you making a fist? Is your face feeling warm? If you are scared, do you feel like shrinking back or running away? Do you feel like the blood is leaving your face? If you are feeling shame or guilt, do you want to hang your head and not look at other people? If you are feeling sad, do you feel like curling up into a ball or sleeping too much? What other things do you feel in your body? Do other people react to your facial expression and ask why you are angry or what is wrong? Sometimes other people may read your emotions better than you do yourself to begin with.

Look over your Impact Statement (pages 47–48) and Stuck Point Log (page 56) and notice how you feel when you say each statement. Look at the Identifying Emotions dia-gram on page 63 to help you identify the name of the emotion you are feeling. Sometimes people have practiced avoiding emotions for so long that it can be hard to know what you feel. If you think to yourself that you don't have any emotion connected to a stuck point, ask yourself, "What would I be feeling if I allowed myself to feel something?" If you're blam-ing yourself, for example, you might feel guilty or ashamed. If you're blaming others, you might feel angry or sad.

Now that you've gotten practice identifying your emotions, the next step is to prac-tice identifying where your emotions are coming from. It's important to tell the difference between an event (a fact like "I was assaulted"), a thought about that fact (for example, "It must have been my fault"), and the emotions that come from that thought (for example, guilt or shame). Just because you say something repeatedly doesn't make it a fact. A fact, like the occurrence of the trauma, is something that happened, not your judgment about it. Your thought is your opinion about what caused the event or what it means. Other people may have different opinions, whereas the facts don't change, unless new evidence or new information emerges. (For example, the fire was not an accident; someone admitted to set-ting it. However, the fact that there was a fire didn't change.)

The next skill, the ABC Worksheet, helps you to notice the connection between events, thoughts, and emotions, first in your day-to-day life and then with the traumatic events that led to your PTSD. The three skills you'll practice with the ABC Worksheet are the follow-ing:

1. Recognize the difference between a fact (an event) and a thought (a stuck point, opinion, or assumption).

2. See which thoughts are connected to the events you experienced, including your traumatic event.

3. Understand what emotions come up when you have those thoughts.

Identifying your thoughts allows you to slow down and consider them carefully, in a way that you might not have before using this book. While some thoughts are accurate and realistic, supported by the facts, it's important to remember that many are not. We all have thoughts pop into our heads that are not completely accurate (for example, "I'll never get this work done" or "This checkout line is taking forever"). However, it's important to remember that thinking something doesn't mean it's true.

How to Complete the ABC Worksheet

The ABC Worksheet on the facing page is a tool to notice the connection between events, thoughts, and emotions. You can also download the ABC Worksheet from *www.guilford.com/resick2-forms* and make copies to fill out electronically or on paper.

In the first column, the A column, you'll write an event. An event is something that happened, whether anyone else witnessed it or not. It is a fact. Examples of facts are "I

ABC Worksheet

A	B	C
Activating event	Belief/stuck point	Consequence
"Something happens"	*"I tell myself something"*	*"I feel something"*

witnessed a murder," "I was in a hurricane," or "I woke up in the hospital." By contrast, a thought, assumption, or opinion is inside your head and cannot be witnessed by anyone else. That would go in the B column instead. Put in the situation that leads you to think the thought in the A column.

The B column is where you'll write your thought. A thought is not the same as a fact or an event. A thought is what you say to yourself about the event, such as an assumption about why it happened. Make sure that what you write down in the B column is a statement, not a question. If your thought is in the form of a question, write down what your answer to that question is currently. For example, if you have been thinking "Why did this happen to me?" you might write your answer to that question, such as "It happened to me because I'm stupid." Later on, you'll learn strategies to evaluate whether the things you say to yourself are accurate and based on facts.

Next, when you think that thought, how do you feel? Put that emotion word in Column C. You can look at the Identifying Emotions diagram on page 63 to help you identify the emotion that goes with the thought you listed in Column B. Don't use emotion words that are too vague, like *bad, upset,* or *bothered.* What is the specific emotion? Emotions are usually one word, like *sad* or *angry.*

If it's a natural feeling that came straight from the event, such as fear in a situation where you were harmed or anger at a perpetrator, those emotions won't last forever but rather lessen over time, and feeling them will help you move toward recovery. So try not to avoid feeling the natural emotions that come up.

However, if your emotion is based on a thought, it might or might not be helpful. For example, you might be feeling guilty if you are thinking "The traumatic event was my fault." It may be one of the reasons you have not recovered from your traumatic event.

First you're learning to identify your thoughts and feelings, and later you'll ask yourself a series of questions to determine if your thought is based on all the facts of what happened. Eventually you may decide that what you've been saying to yourself is not accurate given the context and realities of the traumatic event, but has become a habit of thinking because you heard it or repeated it to yourself many times. You may change what you're saying to yourself to be more balanced. If you do, you'll find that your negative emotions lessen or change completely.

If you want to put more than one event, thought, and feeling on a single worksheet, make sure to draw a line across the paper so that it's clear which event, thought, and feeling go together.

One final note: Sometimes people say "I feel" and then make a statement about how they think. An example would be "I feel I should have done something different." Using the word *feel* in a sentence does not make it an emotion. If you find one of these types of sentences, move it to the B column ("I should have done something different") and then look at the Identifying Emotions diagram on page 63 to decide how you feel about that statement.

The purpose of this chapter is for you to learn that your emotions often follow from what you say to yourself. It makes sense that we feel a certain emotion when we see what we are thinking about a situation. As you work with the ABC Worksheets, you may have to start with C because you notice your emotion first, and then notice what event triggered the emotion and put that in A. Finally, you can focus on what you said to yourself to make you feel that emotion and put that in B.

For example, Gabriela was walking to the store when someone started walking close behind her, and she started to feel scared. She noticed that her heart was racing, her muscles were tensing up, and she started to sweat. Gabriela might write something like the following on her ABC Worksheet, under A, activating event:

I was walking to the store, and someone walked up behind me.

Gabriela knew that she was feeling scared, so she wrote that in the C column, consequence:

Scared

Next, Gabriela needed to figure out what she was saying to herself in that situation that made her feel scared. She asked herself, "What was I thinking then? What made me feel scared?" She wrote the following in the B column, belief/stuck point:

I'm in danger.
Something bad is about to happen.
They're going to hurt me.

So, her final worksheet looked like this:

A	B	C
Activating event "Something happens"	Belief/stuck point "I tell myself something"	Consequence "I feel something"
I was walking to the store, and someone walked up behind me.	I'm in danger. Something bad is about to happen. They're going to hurt me.	Scared

Gabriela filled in this worksheet effectively because she has a fact in the A column, her thoughts about the event in the B column, and her resulting emotion in the C column. It makes sense that Gabriela felt scared given her thought about the meaning of the situation—that she was in danger. Not everyone would feel scared if someone walked up behind them, but they might if they had the same thoughts as Gabriela.

Now you try a practice. Can you think of a time in the last week when you felt a strong emotion, like anger, guilt, or fear? What was going on? What were the facts of the situation? Put that information in A.

A	B	C
Activating event "Something happens"	Belief/stuck point "I tell myself something"	Consequence "I feel something"

If you know what you were thinking, you can put that in B now. Or if you're not sure what you were thinking, you can jump to C. What emotion were you feeling in the situation? Be sure to use an emotion word like those in the Identifying Emotions diagram—for example, *scared, angry,* or *embarrassed.*

Next, ask yourself why you were feeling that emotion in that situation. What were you thinking that made you feel that way? Put that information in B. Try to get all of the thoughts that you were thinking that led to the emotion in C.

Now check: Does the emotion in C match the thought(s) in B? Does it make sense that you felt that emotion given that thought? If not, figure out what else you were saying to yourself that made you feel that emotion. Or is there another emotion that the thoughts in B fueled? If so, add it to the C column.

For example, Lucy initially filled out the following ABC Worksheet:

A	B	C
Activating event "Something happens"	Belief/stuck point "I tell myself something"	Consequence "I feel something"
My daughter had a sports meet, and I couldn't attend.	She wanted me to be there.	Guilty

Lucy thought a little bit more about why it made her feel so guilty that she could not attend her daughter's event when her daughter wanted her to be there. She realized there were more thoughts underneath that first one that led to the guilt, and she added them to her ABC Worksheet:

A	B	C
Activating event "Something happens"	Belief/stuck point "I tell myself something"	Consequence "I feel something"
My daughter had a sports meet, and I couldn't attend.	She really wanted me to be there. I should have been there. I'm a bad mom.	Guilty

It makes sense that Lucy was feeling so guilty—not attending her daughter's sports meet meant to Lucy that she was a bad mom. At least that's what she was telling herself.

> ▶▶| To watch a video to review what you just read here about how to fill out an ABC Worksheet, go to the CPT Whiteboard Video Library (*http://cptforptsd.com/cpt-resources*) and watch the video called *How to Fill Out an ABC Worksheet.* You can also watch a video called *ABC Worksheet Example.*

Do you have any emotions about doing the activities in this book? Do you feel anxious or nervous? If so, that might be a great situation to do an ABC Worksheet on. What are your thoughts about it? For example, you might think something like "I will never get better" or "I can't handle this." If so, it would make sense that you are feeling anxious. In the next chapter you'll have an opportunity to examine your thoughts more closely.

As you practice this skill, you'll get better and better at identifying what thoughts you are having that might be behind your emotions. Most of us are not very aware of our thoughts, so this is really a special skill. Slowing down and identifying your thoughts will also be essential for the next skill, examining what you are saying to yourself, covered in the next chapter.

 PRACTICE ASSIGNMENT ⌇⌇⌇⌇⌇⌇⌇⌇⌇⌇⌇⌇⌇⌇⌇⌇⌇⌇⌇⌇⌇⌇

The next assignment is to practice doing ABC Worksheets. On pages 70–71 you'll find several blank ABC Worksheets you can fill in within the book, and you can also download them from *www.guilford.com/resick2-forms* and make copies to fill out electronically or on paper. Continue to complete ABC Worksheets to become aware of the connections among events, your thoughts, and your feelings. Complete at least one worksheet each day until you feel like you have the hang of it, or for a week. For now, your worksheets can be about everyday events. For example, you could do a worksheet on what you were thinking and feeling when you got cut off in traffic or your friend didn't call when they said they would. Try to fill out the form as soon after an event as possible. That way you'll remember clearly what you were thinking and feeling. Use the Identifying Emotions diagram to help you determine what emotions you are feeling.

 TROUBLESHOOTING ⌇⌇⌇⌇⌇⌇⌇⌇⌇⌇⌇⌇⌇⌇⌇⌇⌇⌇⌇⌇⌇⌇⌇⌇⌇

I don't have feelings. I just feel numb.

Many people with PTSD feel emotionally numb due to avoidance over many years. What about when you have intrusive symptoms? What do you feel then? If you wake up from a nightmare, what are you feeling? Look at the Identifying Emotions diagram again. If you were going to allow yourself to feel your emotions, what would they be? Are you doing something to stop yourself from feeling emotions like drinking, cutting, using drugs, eating to soothe yourself, or smoking? If you stopped those behaviors, what would you feel?

I'm not sure what I am thinking.

Identifying what you are thinking is often the trickiest part. You may have to start with the emotion and ask yourself why you are feeling that way in that situation. What is your best answer? For example, try saying to yourself, "I feel angry because _____
_____."

What you fill in the blank can go in the B column. Practice, practice, practice, and you'll get the hang of it over time!

ABC Worksheets

A	B	C
Activating event	Belief/stuck point	Consequence
"Something happens"	"I tell myself something"	"I feel something"

A	B	C
Activating event	Belief/stuck point	Consequence
"Something happens"	"I tell myself something"	"I feel something"

A	B	C
Activating event	Belief/stuck point	Consequence
"Something happens"	"I tell myself something"	"I feel something"

(continued)

A	B	C
A	**B**	**C**
Activating event	Belief/stuck point	Consequence
"Something happens"	"I tell myself something"	"I feel something"

A	B	C
A	**B**	**C**
Activating event	Belief/stuck point	Consequence
"Something happens"	"I tell myself something"	"I feel something"

A	B	C
A	**B**	**C**
Activating event	Belief/stuck point	Consequence
"Something happens"	"I tell myself something"	"I feel something"

A	B	C
A	**B**	**C**
Activating event	Belief/stuck point	Consequence
"Something happens"	"I tell myself something"	"I feel something"

Reviewing the ABC Worksheet and Applying It to Your Trauma

In this chapter, you learned how to use the ABC Worksheet. Look over your completed ABC Worksheets and ask yourself if you were able to get a factual event into the A column (just a few words), the thought about that event in the B column (like stuck points on your Stuck Point Log), and a single word in the C column to describe your emotion when you think that thought. Also reflect on whether the emotions match the thoughts in B. Did you figure out what you were thinking that made you feel those emotions? If you did, give yourself a pat on the back. Well done!

Please notice if you had a range of emotions over the course of going through the ABC Worksheets or if there were patterns in the kinds of thoughts and emotions you experienced. Do you tend to get angry at yourself or others? If this is the case, it's possible that you have an underlying stuck point that you may have had much of your life, like "I can't do anything right" or "No one can be trusted." We call this a **core belief,** a way of thinking that you have had so long, perhaps since childhood, that you don't even have to think about it anymore. You just accept it as fact and move on to being angry at yourself or others (or depressed). Keep an eye out for stuck points that come up over and over again in different situations, directed at either yourself or others. If you noticed any thoughts like those that aren't yet on your Stuck Point Log (page 56), add them now.

Great work applying this new skill to your everyday situations. You're building a special skill to identify the thoughts that drive your emotions. Next, you'll apply this skill to your index trauma.

Applying the ABC Worksheet to the Traumatic Event

Now you can apply the same ABC skill to your traumatic experience and your thoughts about why it happened. Just as you did for the everyday events, identify your thoughts and the emotions that are connected to those thoughts.

Start by putting your index trauma in Column A. Just a few words will do, like "Sexual abuse by my cousin when I was nine," "Witnessed my friend being shot," or "I was hit by a car."

A	B	C
Activating event "Something happens"	Belief/stuck point "I tell myself something"	Consequence "I feel something"

Next, write in a thought you have about the traumatic event. You can refer to your Stuck Point Log (page 56) for this. In particular, do you have any stuck points on your log about why the trauma happened, who was to blame for it, or ways that it could have been prevented? For example, "I should have done _____" or "If only I had done _____, the event would not have happened." If so, start by putting one of these thoughts in the B column.

Finally, consider what emotion you feel when you think that thought. Write that under C. Often people feel guilt, shame, regret, or anger at themselves when they think thoughts about what they "should have" done.

Here is an example from Joseph, whose brother died by a drug overdose:

A	B	C
Activating event "Something happens"	Belief/stuck point "I tell myself something"	Consequence "I feel something"
My brother's overdose	I should have done more to help him	Guilty

This activity will help you see where some of your strong negative emotions about the trauma may be coming from. It makes sense that Joseph has been feeling guilty given that he has been taking on some of the blame for his brother's overdose, thinking that he should have done more to prevent it. In the next chapter, you'll be able to take a closer look at what you've been saying to yourself to see if it is helpful and realistic.

As you write down your emotions on your ABC Worksheet, remember that there are two kinds of feelings: those that arise from the event itself and the kind that arise from what you tell yourself about the event. If it's a natural emotion that came straight from the event, such as fear in the situation where you were harmed, sadness at losses, or anger at a perpetrator, feeling those emotions will help you move toward recovery. They won't last forever and will become less intense over time. Natural emotions are like the bubbles in a soda bottle. The contents are under pressure when the lid is on, and while they might come out strongly when you first open it up, the contents soon settle down. Natural emotions are the same way. If you've been pushing them down, when you first allow yourself to feel them, they can feel quite strong. But after you experience them, you'll notice that they begin to decrease and you'll start to feel differently. This is the process of recovery. You acknowledge the weight of what happened, and you allow yourself to feel it. The memory will remain, but the feelings that go with it won't be as intense after you have processed them. So try not to avoid feeling natural emotions. They won't be as intense forever. At some point you might feel them in passing when you encounter a reminder, but the reminders won't hold the same power to trigger the really strong emotions.

Other emotions are based on thoughts or interpretations of events. For example, you might be feeling guilty if you're thinking "The traumatic event was my fault." Or you may be angry with yourself if you're thinking "I never should have left the house that night.

I should have trusted my gut." Those thoughts may be one of the reasons you have not recovered from your traumatic event. Joseph's guilt is an example of a manufactured emotion because it is coming from his thought about what he "should have" done differently. Eventually if you decide what you have been saying to yourself is not accurate given the context and realities of the traumatic event, you may change what you're saying to yourself to be more balanced, and most likely you'll find that your manufactured emotions lessen or change completely.

Before moving on, did you complete an ABC Worksheet on your worst traumatic event? Or did you avoid or skip over it? If you haven't done it yet, go back and do it now. This is essential to the next step of the program.

Mark didn't do an ABC Worksheet on his index event and chose instead to do a worksheet on a different, less distressing event in his life. He realized that he was avoiding feeling the shame that was involved in the index event and went back and did another ABC Worksheet on the worst event. By the time he reread the ABC Worksheet on that event and saw it on the page, he started to realize that it was not his shame to own, but that of his perpetrator.

If you are still having a hard time getting yourself to do a worksheet on the most distressing traumatic event, notice whether you have a stuck point about doing an ABC Worksheet and, if so, do a worksheet on that stuck point (for example, A = doing an ABC Worksheet on my worst trauma; B = "If I write it down, that will make the trauma real"; C = scared). Don't delay. You've come this far, so don't turn back now! Often people start to feel better after the next chapter. So, do an ABC Worksheet on your index trauma, and then as soon as you've done that, continue to the next chapter.

*   *   *

Keep tracking your symptoms each week using the Graph for Tracking Your Weekly Scores on page 24. After this next chapter, you may start to notice a change in your symptoms if you haven't already.

Complete the PTSD Checklist to track your symptoms as you complete this book. Be sure to complete this measure on the same index event each time. When the instructions and questions refer to a "stressful experience," remember that that is your index event—the worst event that you are working on first.

Write in here the trauma that you are working on first: _____

Complete this PTSD Checklist with reference to that event.

Instructions: Below is a list of problems that people sometimes have in response to a very stressful experience. Please read each problem carefully, and then circle one of the numbers to the right to indicate how much you have been bothered by that problem *in the past week*.

In the past week, how much were you bothered by:	Not at all	A little bit	Mod- erately	Quite a bit	Extremely
1. Repeated, disturbing, and unwanted memories of the stressful experience?	0	1	2	3	4
2. Repeated, disturbing dreams of the stressful experience?	0	1	2	3	4
3. Suddenly feeling or acting as if the stressful experience were actually happening again (*as if you were actually back there reliving it*)?	0	1	2	3	4
4. Feeling very upset when something reminded you of the stressful experience?	0	1	2	3	4
5. Having strong physical reactions when something reminded you of the stressful experience (*for example, heart pounding, trouble breathing, sweating*)?	0	1	2	3	4
6. Avoiding memories, thoughts, or feelings related to the stressful experience?	0	1	2	3	4
7. Avoiding external reminders of the stressful experience (*for example, people, places, conversations, activities, objects, or situations*)?	0	1	2	3	4
8. Trouble remembering important parts of the stressful experience (not due to head injury or substances)?	0	1	2	3	4
9. Having strong negative beliefs about yourself, other people, or the world (*for example, having thoughts such as I am bad, There is something seriously wrong with me, No one can be trusted, or The world is completely dangerous*)?	0	1	2	3	4
10. Blaming yourself or someone else (who didn't intend the outcome) for the stressful experience or what happened after it?	0	1	2	3	4
11. Having strong negative feelings, such as fear, horror, anger, guilt, or shame?	0	1	2	3	4
12. Loss of interest in activities that you used to enjoy?	0	1	2	3	4
13. Feeling distant or cut off from other people?	0	1	2	3	4
14. Trouble experiencing positive feelings (*for example, being unable to feel happiness or have loving feelings for people close to you*)?	0	1	2	3	4
15. Irritable behavior, angry outbursts, or acting aggressively?	0	1	2	3	4
16. Taking too many risks or doing things that could cause you harm?	0	1	2	3	4
17. Being "super alert" or watchful or on guard?	0	1	2	3	4
18. Feeling jumpy or easily startled?	0	1	2	3	4
19. Having difficulty concentrating?	0	1	2	3	4
20. Trouble falling or staying asleep?	0	1	2	3	4

Add up the total and write it here: _____

Part III

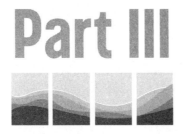

Getting Unstuck from Beliefs about the Trauma

By now, you've had the chance to look at the connections between your thoughts and your emotions. This is an important step, and it doesn't come naturally for everyone, but taking the time to consider your own thoughts and feelings has helped prepare you for the next step. Hopefully, you were able to see that the strong emotions that you have been feeling make sense and are not coming out of nowhere. Your emotions are influenced by your thoughts and interpretations. So, if you've been blaming yourself for your trauma or what happened after it, it's no wonder you have been feeling guilty or ashamed. If you've been thinking the world is completely dangerous and people will always hurt you, it makes sense that you've been feeling scared and anxious.

It's also worth commending yourself for having taken a big step by completing an ABC Worksheet on your index trauma. Avoidance is a symptom of PTSD, and it can be hard to think about your worst event. So congratulations for not avoiding! You are setting yourself up for success in recovering from PTSD.

Now that you have taken the time to figure out what stuck points might be getting in the way of your recovery, you're ready to start applying some skills to your thinking about the trauma. In the next chapter, you'll learn to ask yourself questions to examine the facts about the trauma. This process can help you look at any stuck points you may have about the cause of the trauma. Then you'll have the opportunity to use a series of worksheets to help you master the skill of examining your thoughts. Most people start feeling better once they work through this part of the process, so keep up the good work, and let's get started!

Beginning to Examine Your Worst Traumatic Event

Now that you have learned the ABC skill, you'll be able to start to examine some of your thoughts about the traumatic event. It's important to ask yourself questions like the ones we ask below about your thoughts about *why* the trauma happened. These questions are intended to help you look at the whole picture, without leaving anything out, and look at it in different ways to see whether your beliefs are balanced, accurate, and a fair assessment of what actually happened.

People often have thoughts that they "should" or "shouldn't" have done something related to their trauma. Do you have any thoughts like these? If so, it's important to remember what the reasons were that you did the things you did, and didn't do something different. People often have a logical reason for making the choices they made, or they didn't really have a choice at all. It's important to remember what the context was for you: What did you know then? How old were you? How were you feeling? How much control did you have? These facts may help you make sense of why you did what you did and didn't take different actions.

If you have been questioning things that you did regarding your index trauma, what were the reasons you did what you did? (For example, if you've been thinking to yourself "I shouldn't have gone out that night," what are the reasons you decided to go out?)

_____

_____

_____

_____

If you've been questioning things you did *not* do, what were the reasons you didn't take different action? (For example, if you've been thinking "I should have told someone about the abuse," why didn't you at the time?)

_____

_____

_____

_____

It's also essential to remember what the context was at the time. It's important to consider the whole story of what happened. Don't forget about the impact that a fight–flight–freeze response may have had or about what was actually possible in the moment that the event(s) occurred. What were you thinking and feeling at the time?

_____

_____

_____

_____

How old were you, and what was your state of mind at the time?

_____

_____

_____

Did you have full control of the situation?

_____

_____

_____

_____

Let's look at how Julian answered these questions about a time that he was jumped when he was walking home one night. His thought was "I never should have gone out that night." When reflecting on these questions, he realized that he went out because his friend invited him over. While he knew that there was some risk going out at night because there was sometimes violence in his neighborhood, he also wanted to see his friend and relax after a busy week and didn't think he would be the victim of a crime. He also believed "I should have fought back." He went through the preceding questions and realized that he was surprised and afraid at the time, that he had a freeze response (which is an automatic response to danger), and that there were several men who were larger than he was. He didn't know if they had weapons with them and thought that fighting could have ended up with his getting hurt even worse. Also, he sustained a blow to the head and was too injured to put up much of a fight after that. Remembering these facts helped Julian move from anger at himself to a feeling of compassion for himself. He had tried to do the best he could to survive in a situation that took him by surprise and that he couldn't control.

Considering Your Role in an Event

When thinking about blame and responsibility for an event, it's important to consider the specific role that each person played. In society, laws and courts assign different consequences based on an individual's level of control and intent in a situation. When thinking about your traumatic experience, consider **the role that you and others played**. When deciding how much responsibility or blame to give to individuals, it's important to consider **how much they knew** and **how much control they had**. The diagram below illustrates this.

Your Role in the Traumatic Event: What Are the Facts?

In the first case, the traumatic event would be something **unforeseeable or uncontrollable**. For example, if you were driving and your car ran over something, blew a tire, spun out, and hit another car, you couldn't have foreseen that. You had no way of knowing the tire would blow right in that moment. You would have no blame and would not be charged with a crime. Although you might be traumatized by the event, you would not have caused it or been able to foresee it or stop it. It was a surprise to you and/or out of

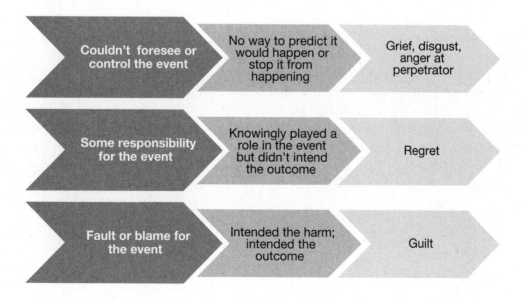

your control. In this case, it would be appropriate to have natural emotions like fear, anger, grief, or sadness.

Thinking about your worst traumatic event, did you know that that exact event would happen that day?

_____

Did you have full control over the event?

_____

If you answered "No" to either of the above, then the event was unforeseeable/uncontrollable, and it would be going overboard to say that the event was your "responsibility" or "fault" or to feel regret or guilt over it.

The second case would apply if you had some **responsibility** for the event (for example, if you got into a collision when you were speeding and texting). However, if you didn't *intend* to harm anyone, it would make sense to have regret that it happened, and you might even be charged for a crime because you were speeding or texting, but the sentence would not be as severe as if you did have intent. (For example, U.S. law differentiates between manslaughter—no intent to kill or harm—and murder, which involves intent to kill.)

Maybe you are thinking that you played a role in the event, but really it was unavoidable (like walking alone at night in a neighborhood that you knew was dangerous after your car broke down, or not being old enough to understand the consequences of your behavior). In this situation, your natural emotion might be sadness that it happened or anger that someone hurt you. It still might be considered unforeseeable or uncontrollable. Things can still be unforeseeable if the risk is not zero, or if something is possible but usually doesn't happen. For example, if you live in an area where there are occasional muggings or assaults but they are low in frequency and don't occur on most days, you could not have foreseen that it would happen to you at the exact time that it did—even if you knew it was possible that it could happen in the area where you live. **If you had truly been able to foresee it, you probably would have tried to avoid it.**

Only in the final case that you see in the diagram on page 81 would we use the terms *fault* or *blame,* because there was a clear intention to do harm. If someone intends to hurt someone else, then guilt may be an appropriate emotion. Looking back at the particular traumatic event that you decided to work on first, ask yourself whether you intended the outcome.

Did you intend for the outcome that occurred to happen?

_____

What was your intent? What did you assume would happen that day?

_____

_____

_____

_____

If you were in a similar situation before, what occurred then and what were your expectations this time?

_____

_____

_____

_____

If you didn't intend the outcome but you did something that you knew could cause something bad to happen (for example, driving drunk), you may have some regrets. Regret would be an appropriate reaction in a situation like this. However, you can still come to terms with the fact that you didn't _intend_ to harm anyone, and it doesn't have to define who you are for the rest of your life. Anyone can make mistakes or do things they wish they hadn't. No one is perfect, and people learn and change from their experiences.

If you _did_ intend for the event to occur (for example, you hurt someone on purpose), then you may experience guilt—and it may be understandable that you feel guilt over your actions. You may need to think through what happened to determine if there were any factors that played a role in why you decided to do what you did (for example, if you didn't have other good options and the action you took seemed to be the best way to escape the situation or remain alive, to save someone else, or to sustain less harm). If you did intend the outcome and there are no other facts that you have left out of the situation, then guilt may be the appropriate emotion. Then you'll have to put the event into the context of your whole life, before and after. Are you the same person now who you were then? Have you continued harming people intentionally? Did this happen at a time when you were in extreme and difficult circumstances? Can you find ways to give back to your community to make up for any harm you've done? Are you living differently and making different decisions now?

In his youth, Richard sold drugs for a living. One night he got into an altercation and shot someone when the situation escalated out of control. He believed that he had no other choice if he didn't want to be hurt or even killed. He served time in prison, and when he got out, he was clean and sober and decided not to go back to his old neighborhood and got a job in a factory instead. He still experiences guilt about his decision to shoot the man. He sent a letter of apology to the man's family and began volunteering with a local organization that works with justice-involved youth, hoping that his story could help others decide to take a different path. Richard worked to contextualize the shooting within the bigger picture of his life and who he is now, and is focused on moving forward and living a life he feels proud of now.

Hindsight Bias

People like to think they can predict the future and often say that they "should have known" that their trauma was going to happen, but was it actually predictable that the event would unfold the way it did, at the time that it did? We sometimes think with **hindsight bias** by looking back, judging past actions based on what we know now, after the fact—that is, sometimes people overestimate their ability to have predicted an outcome that could not possibly have been foreseen.

Consider the following questions:

Did you know then exactly what was going to happen and when, or is this a case of hindsight?

_____

_____

_____

_____

Are you imagining that if something had been changed, the outcome would have been better?

_____

Is it possible that the event might have happened anyway, or even been worse if you'd done something different? How so?

_____

_____

_____

_____

Were you doing things that you had done before or since without a bad outcome? Describe.

_____

_____

_____

_____

Have other people you know done the same things without having a bad outcome?

_____

_____

_____

_____

What did you intend to happen by doing what you did (or by not doing something else)?

_____

_____

_____

_____

Was there really anything you realistically could have done to stop or prevent the event? Consider not what you think now but what you knew at the time that it occurred, how fast it happened, what skills you had, and what options you considered *at the time*.

_____

_____

_____

_____

Anything you thought of later or wish you could have done doesn't count. It wasn't an option if you didn't think of it or couldn't do it then. And if you did have options, was there a reason you chose the one(s) you did?

_____

_____

_____

_____

Is it possible that the outcome might have been worse if you hadn't chosen that option?

_____

_____

_____

_____

In hindsight, you may think of many other things you wish you could have done, but it's important to think about the circumstances at the time. Could you have actually done them? Are you second-guessing yourself unfairly? It isn't realistic to try to undo the event after it happens by second-guessing yourself with what you know now that you didn't know then. Before it happened, you were unlikely to know what was coming.

If you are still feeling stuck, answer some more questions about the event like the following:

Who else was there or involved?

_____

_____

_____

_____

Did other people play a role in the event?

_____

_____

_____

_____

Did others have intention to harm you or someone else? What decisions did they make at the time?

_____

_____

_____

_____

What options did you really have then, if any? Did you have any good options that you knew of or only bad options or no options?

_____

_____

_____

_____

Why did you make the choices you did, if in fact you made any choices at all?

_____

_____

_____

_____

What facts or details are you leaving out when you remember what happened? Are you forgetting to give responsibility or blame to anyone else? Are you minimizing what you did do to help yourself or others? Are you exaggerating how much control you had?

_____

_____

_____

_____

It can also be helpful to consider whether you are focused on just one piece of why the event happened and leaving out other key details; see the diagram below as an example.

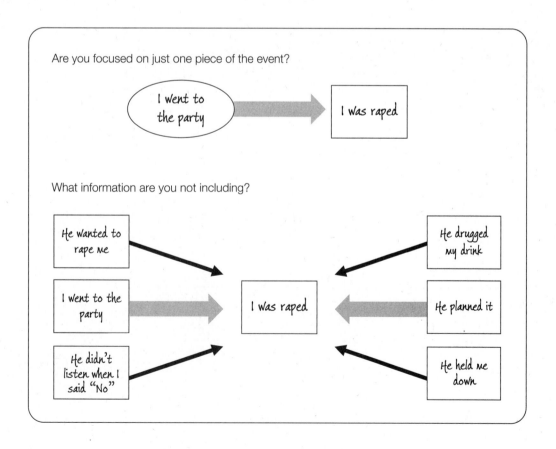

Questions to consider:

How much responsibility are you giving to this one factor? For example, how much are you thinking that the trauma happened because of something about you or because of something you did or didn't do?

_____

_____

_____

_____

What other factors were involved?

_____

_____

_____

_____

Which is the best explanation for why the event happened? What was the most direct cause? Who had the intent?

_____

_____

_____

_____

Take a moment to reflect on what you are thinking now about your role in the trauma. As you consider the facts of the event, including what the context was and others' roles in it, is your thinking about your role in the trauma shifting in any way? If you were originally blaming yourself, thinking it was your fault, or that you "should have" done something differently, are you starting to notice any other ways of thinking about the situation? If so, how does it feel to think about the trauma differently?

_____

_____

_____

_____

This is important and difficult work, so we commend you on the efforts you're putting in to think through the facts of the trauma and start to examine your stuck points. Don't worry if you're still struggling with guilt or self-blame. You're still at the beginning of this process, and examining your thoughts is a new skill. If you've been avoiding thinking about the trauma until now, this may be the first time in a long time that you're revisiting the facts. Stuck points can become habits over time, and changing our thinking takes time. Be patient with yourself and continue in the process to try additional strategies to help get you unstuck.

Examining the Role of Others

Sometimes people know, or begin to realize, that the trauma was not their fault, and some of their stuck points focus on the role of others. Is it possible that you are blaming someone who didn't intend the harm and avoiding thinking about the actual perpetrator (for example, "My mother should have known that my uncle was abusing me when he stayed with me while she was at work. I was too scared to tell her, but she should have been able to tell" or "My friends should have been looking out for me at the party" and "If they hadn't left me alone with him, it wouldn't have happened"). A common example is when someone who was physically or sexually abused as a child finds themselves blaming one of their parents for not protecting them ("She shouldn't have left me alone with him" or "My mom should have left my abusive father instead of letting him hurt us"). Combat veterans may also find themselves with stuck points, such as "They never should have sent us out on that mission." In these situations, it's important to consider the information you are leaving out.

What was the context? What information and resources were available to those individuals at the time?

_____
_____
_____
_____

What other factors may have influenced what happened?

_____
_____
_____
_____

Who else bears responsibility or blame for what happened?

_____
_____
_____
_____

Who had the intent to harm?

_____

_____

_____

_____

In circumstances when others did not protect you from harm, it can be helpful to consider the following questions:

Were there other factors at play? For example, was that person also abused or intimidated, or were they in danger, too?

_____

_____

_____

_____

If they were also in a dangerous situation, did they realistically have the means to remove you and themselves from the situation? What factors might have been in the way?

_____

_____

_____

_____

If you have stuck points, such as "They should have known what was happening/what would happen," think back to what information was available to them. Was the event something they could have reasonably anticipated? Was there a high chance it would happen?

_____

_____

_____

_____

How much responsibility should be assigned to anyone other than the person who decided to do the harm versus someone who might have protected you?

_____

_____

_____

_____

_____

If the trauma was a form of abuse that happened decades ago or in a different place, were there the same resources and knowledge about child abuse or interpersonal violence that are available now? Did they have the means and support to change the situation?

_____

_____

_____

_____

If they did know and didn't do anything, or enough, to stop the abuse, consider what types of support they had, social values that may have existed (for example, "sweep it under the rug," "What happens in the family is their business"), and their own knowledge and capabilities. What do you conclude about their reaction?

_____

_____

_____

_____

If the abuser groomed you, did they also groom others to look the other way, not ask questions, or did they intimidate or threaten them? Were they in a position of power over others?

_____

_____

_____

_____

Who else has responsibility or blame for what happened? Are you minimizing the role of a direct perpetrator? Who actually had the intent to harm?

_____

_____

_____

_____

These factors may need to be considered, not to make excuses for people who may have been in a position to protect you but to consider the broader context—just as you do for your consideration of stuck points about what you should/could have done differently.

It can also help to portion out responsibility based on the facts of the situation. For example, if you have been thinking that your mother is to blame for not stopping sexual abuse by another family member, key facts may be what she knew when. If you're not one hundred percent sure that she knew the abuse was going on, it might have been unforeseeable to her, too, at that point. If you eventually told her you were being abused and she didn't take any actions to stop the abuse and it continued, then it would make sense to give her some responsibility for the abuse. After all, you did the really hard task of telling someone what was happening, and she failed to act to protect you. However, considering the other factors may help you understand her actions, even if they are not excusable or acceptable.

Likewise, if you are a veteran, you may blame others for things that they didn't directly cause related to combat. For example, if you are blaming leadership for sending you or others on a mission where there was an enemy attack, it can be helpful to consider who really intended the harm—leadership or the enemy combatants—and portion out blame and responsibility accordingly. If command was truly negligent, they might have some responsibility, but considering the context and who took the steps to harm you or others would be key.

Continuing to Use the ABC Worksheets

Over the next days, continue to use the ABC Worksheets (pages 95–98) to look at thoughts from your Stuck Point Log (page 56) about why the index trauma happened. As you do your ABC Worksheets each day, consider the questions from this chapter when you look at your stuck points in the B column.

Now that you are evaluating some of your thinking, you may be able to practice coming up with alternative ways of thinking about the event. On this next version of the ABC Worksheet, try filling in an additional part of the worksheet. The first question is whether the thought in B is realistic. In other words, do you know with one hundred percent certainty that what is written in the B column is a fact, or could there be other ways of looking at it? Another question to ask yourself is whether the thought in B is helpful. If your stuck point is not realistic or not helpful, then answer the next question: What can you tell yourself on such occasions in the future? In other words, if the thought in B is not a fact or is not helpful to keep thinking, what would be a more helpful thing to say? For example, instead of "The abuse was my fault," you might decide that "The abuse was my abuser's fault."

Here is an example:

A	B	C
Activating event "Something happens"	Belief/stuck point "I tell myself something"	Consequence "I feel something"
I was assaulted as part of a hate crime	I should have known not to go to that part of town	Angry at myself

Are my thoughts above in B *realistic or helpful?*   No, it's not helpful to blame myself.

What can you tell yourself on such occasions in the future? *I didn't know the assault would happen. My actions did not cause the assault. The perpetrators are the ones at fault. They are the ones who chose to hurt me.*

✎ PRACTICE ASSIGNMENT

Use the ABC Worksheet (Full Version) at the bottom of this page to become aware of the connection among events, thoughts, and feelings. You can also download and make extra copies of this version of the ABC Worksheet from *www.guilford.com/resick2-forms*. Then, continue to complete at least one worksheet each day until you have worked on all of your stuck points about why the trauma happened, or for a week. You can find more ABC Worksheets on pages 95–98. Complete **all** of the worksheets about the worst traumatic event (beliefs like "I should have done _____" and "It's my fault"). Continue to use the Identifying Emotions diagram on page 63 to help you determine what emotions you are feeling, and try to complete the questions at the

ABC Worksheet (Full Version)

A Activating event *"Something happens"*	B Belief/stuck point *"I tell myself something"*	C Consequence *"I feel something"*

Are my thoughts above in B *realistic* or *helpful*? _____

What can you tell yourself on such occasions in the future?

_____

_____

bottom of each ABC Worksheet if you can see other ways of looking at the event using the questions in this chapter.

Sometimes people want to avoid at this point but you are potentially very close to making important changes in your thinking that may make you feel significantly better, so keep at it! You can do this!

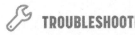 TROUBLESHOOTING

Can I do the ABC Worksheets on other traumas instead? Why do I have to stick to one?

It's best to stick to the index event for now. You are learning skills that will help you reevaluate your stuck points, working a little each day on the event that causes you the most PTSD symptoms. It may seem easier to work on another trauma or life event first, but it's important to start with the one that gives you the most PTSD symptoms because that in turn will make working on the other events easier. Jumping from event to event might slow your progress. If you work a little bit on the index trauma, then jump to another trauma, it doesn't give you as much of a chance to fully work through the index trauma. In fact, deciding to work on another trauma that is not quite as difficult to think about can be a way to avoid thinking about and remembering the index trauma. If you believe you've made good progress on your index trauma and you no longer believe some of the things you've told yourself about why it happened, that's wonderful! Sticking with it a little longer can help you continue to consolidate those gains. Later in the program, once you have worked through your stuck points about the index event more fully, you can apply the skills to stuck points you have about other traumas.

I notice I feel worse when I am doing the worksheets. I feel the urge to avoid by doing things that are unhelpful (drinking, cutting).

Intense feelings mean you are no longer avoiding, which is an important step in your recovery. It's a good thing, not bad, if you are finally feeling natural emotions, like sadness that it happened, how terrified you were, or anger at a perpetrator. It's tempting to avoid and to pursue your go-to (but unhelpful and potentially harmful) avoidance and coping habits. Remember that the intensity of your natural emotions is temporary. Reach out to someone who is supportive and helpful and let them know you are struggling, or substitute a healthier coping strategy (exercise, reading, or watching something you enjoy), as long as you give yourself some time to feel the emotions as well.

For example, whenever Cynthia spent time working on the ABC Worksheets, she noticed that she wanted to pour herself a glass of wine. She knew that this would help her numb out and make the feelings less intense, and this was her go-to avoidance strategy. Cynthia decided to put the wine she had in her house into a box in the garage so it would be harder to go on "autopilot" and pour herself a glass. She planned some activities she could do right after she did her worksheets. Some days she met up with a supportive friend to take a walk. Other days she decided to work on a craft project or pull some weeds in her yard.

A	B	C
Activating event	Belief/stuck point	Consequence
"Something happens"	*"I tell myself something"*	*"I feel something"*

Are my thoughts above in B *realistic* or *helpful?* _____

What can you tell yourself on such occasions in the future?

_____

_____

A	B	C
Activating event	Belief/stuck point	Consequence
"Something happens"	*"I tell myself something"*	*"I feel something"*

Are my thoughts above in B *realistic* or *helpful?* _____

What can you tell yourself on such occasions in the future?

_____

_____

(continued)

A Activating event *"Something happens"*	**B** Belief/stuck point *"I tell myself something"*	**C** Consequence *"I feel something"*

Are my thoughts above in B *realistic* or *helpful?* _____

What can you tell yourself on such occasions in the future?

_____

_____

A Activating event *"Something happens"*	**B** Belief/stuck point *"I tell myself something"*	**C** Consequence *"I feel something"*

Are my thoughts above in B *realistic* or *helpful?* _____

What can you tell yourself on such occasions in the future?

_____

_____

(continued)

ABC Worksheets (Full Version) *(page 3 of 4)*

A Activating event "Something happens"	B Belief/stuck point "I tell myself something"	C Consequence "I feel something"

Are my thoughts above in B *realistic* or *helpful*? _____

What can you tell yourself on such occasions in the future?

_____

_____

A Activating event "Something happens"	B Belief/stuck point "I tell myself something"	C Consequence "I feel something"

Are my thoughts above in B *realistic* or *helpful*? _____

What can you tell yourself on such occasions in the future?

_____

_____

(continued)

A	B	C
Activating event	Belief/stuck point	Consequence
"Something happens"	"I tell myself something"	"I feel something"

Are my thoughts above in B *realistic* or *helpful?* _____

What can you tell yourself on such occasions in the future?

_____

_____

These activities allowed her some time to feel the emotions that the worksheets brought up, but then she noticed that her attention shifted back to what she was doing in the moment. Soon it got easier to do the worksheets without turning to a glass of wine.

If you are feeling manufactured emotions like guilt and shame due to hindsight bias or blaming yourself for something you could not have realistically controlled, that is exactly why you are being asked to fill out the worksheets. Refer to the questions in this chapter to help you look more closely at the thoughts behind those emotions. Do you notice when you look at the facts that your emotions change? Once you process and resolve your index event, you may notice that your distress begins to decrease.

I am getting irritable, and my family and friends have said if it's making me feel upset, maybe I should quit.

Are you irritable because you are feeling natural emotions, or are you frustrated because it's difficult to face what you have been thinking and feeling about your index event? Explain to your family that you are experiencing emotions that you have avoided ever since the traumas happened, but that they are temporary. Irritable behavior is actually a symptom of PTSD, and you're working on reducing PTSD right now. It can help to explain the rationale for this approach to people close to you and ask for their support to face the trauma instead of avoiding. Giving them some information about PTSD may help them know how to support you. The National Center for PTSD whiteboard video *What Is PTSD?* (*https://bit.ly/3zsRvTL*) you watched in Chapter 4 might be a good thing to show them, and you can give them the handout called "Supporting Your Loved One During CPT" in the Appendix.

I see what you mean with all the questions you asked in this chapter, but I still feel like the traumatic event is my fault.

You are just getting started looking at your thoughts, so it is absolutely OK if you still feel like your stuck points are true. You'll have a lot more opportunities to keep examining the evidence over the coming weeks. As you go along, if you are still feeling stuck, it could help to think about the following: Why must it be your fault? Why is it important that you hang on to the idea that it must be your fault? What would it mean if it was unforeseeable or someone else had the intent (and fault and blame)? Is that a scary idea? Does it mean that you don't have complete control over future events? Unfortunately, none of us do. We all have some control, but not total control. (You'll work more on these topics later in the book.) Would it mean something scary or difficult to accept about a perpetrator whose role you've previously minimized if you acknowledged their role and responsibility for what happened? Your answers to these questions might suggest additional thoughts to add to your Stuck Point Log and work on next.

What if I know that the trauma wasn't my fault?

It's great if the work you've done has brought you to a point of understanding that your trauma was not your fault. Or maybe you've always known that on some level, even if it "feels like" it was. The question to ask yourself then is "Why is the event still haunting me?" Look at your symptoms on the PTSD Checklist and ask yourself why you have them. Do you have a just-world stuck point about fairness, such as "Things like this aren't supposed to happen" or "It's not fair that this happened to me"? If you are feeling strong emotions related to the situation you wrote down in A, ask yourself why you are so angry (or sad, humiliated, scared, etc.). Try filling in the blank: "I'm feeling [emotion] because

_____

_____."

The answer is the thought to write in the B column. Even if you don't have a stuck point about self-blame, you can complete an ABC Worksheet on the event. Maybe you feel a natural emotion related to the event. Have you let yourself experience the natural emotions? What's keeping you from doing that? There might be a stuck point like "If I let myself feel grief and sadness about what happened, I won't be able to handle it" or "If I let myself acknowledge and feel the fear I experienced during the trauma, I'll totally fall apart." If so, add these to your Stuck Point Log. You'll be learning tools to address those stuck points over the next few chapters.

Reviewing Your ABC Worksheets

How did completing the full version of the ABC Worksheets on the traumatic experience go? Were you able to complete the bottom portion of the worksheet and see any other ways of looking at the situation? If you had trouble with this, refer back to the last section to consider the context, what you knew at the time, how much control you had, and what your intention was. See if you can find anything more factual to say, even if you don't believe it one hundred percent right now.

~~~~~ Beliefs about Fairness ~~~~~

Perhaps some of your stuck points are about fairness—for example, "Things like this aren't supposed to happen to innocent children," or "I must have done something to deserve it." Remember that these kinds of thoughts are examples of the just-world belief, the idea that the world is just or fair. Because most of us were taught to think this way, when something goes wrong, our first instinct might be to figure out what we did wrong to cause it, assuming that bad things happen (as punishment) only when you've done something "wrong" or been "bad." Or we might have beliefs about how the world is "supposed" to work, assuming things are fair.

If you've done an ABC Worksheet on a just-world belief like "It happened as punishment" or "I must have been bad," or if you have any stuck points on your log like these, consider the following:

Is the belief, or what it implies, always the case? For example, do people always get what they deserve? Is life always fair?

_____
_____
_____
_____

What exceptions can you think of? Consider, for example, things you've heard from other people or stories you've heard reported in the media.

_____
_____
_____
_____

If you're thinking you did something to deserve what happened . . . what did you do to deserve it? (Your answer below might be something to put on the Stuck Point Log, page 56, to consider more carefully.)

_____

_____

_____

_____

Is the outcome you experienced *always* the consequence when people do what you did? Can you list any exceptions?

_____

_____

_____

_____

Does the "punishment fit the 'crime'"? Does that seem like a reasonable consequence for what you did or didn't do? Explain why or why not.

_____

_____

_____

_____

Are there any other possible explanations for why the trauma happened?

_____

_____

_____

_____

On the topic of fairness, please keep in mind that justice does not exist in nature. If you've ever watched a nature show, you've probably already learned as much. For example, animals kill other animals. That may be "fair" for the animal that needs to eat, but it doesn't seem "fair" to the animal that was killed. As humans, we set up rules and laws in an attempt to get people to behave in ways that won't harm one another. Sometimes it works and sometimes it doesn't, because people have free will and can disobey laws. Sometimes traumas don't happen for a "good reason." They just happen. The world is not naturally fair, but sometimes we are lucky and sometimes we are not. You don't always get a ticket if you speed, but sometimes you do. And sometimes you aren't doing anything wrong but something terrible happens anyway.

~~~~~~~~ Noticing Changes in Emotions ~~~~~~~~

If you were able to reconsider any of your stuck points, what did you notice happening with your emotions? Did they change at all? Often when we change what we say to ourselves, our emotions also change.

Adina's husband assaulted her in front of their daughter. Originally, she was think-ing to herself "I shouldn't have provoked him. It's my fault my daughter saw him hit me." These thoughts made her feel ashamed. Nonetheless, Adina used the skills in the last section, particularly considering what her intention was, examining for hindsight, and identifying other factors.

Intention. Adina concluded the following: "It wasn't my intent to be hit or to make my husband angry. My intention was to ask my husband a question to help our daughter."

Hindsight. Adina reflected that her thought that she "shouldn't have pro-voked" her husband by asking him a question was hindsight because she was look-ing back, questioning her actions based on what she now knows happened after-ward. However, at the time she didn't know her husband would assault her. In fact, he had never assaulted her in front of their daughter before. She also realized that even if she hadn't asked him a question then, he might have assaulted her in front of their daughter anyhow because of the mood he was in that day, or at another time. As she recalled, he would fly off the handle unexpectedly at times, and she couldn't predict when it would happen.

Considering other factors. Adina also realized that she was focusing on just one factor in her thinking about the trauma—that she had asked a question that "provoked" her husband. However, she realized that this was not the only factor. Lots of women ask their husbands questions and do not get assaulted. What caused her assault was that her husband chose to assault her. When she considered her hus-band's role in the assault, she took the responsibility off herself. She recognized that other couples have disagreements and ask each other questions without abuse, so it wasn't fair to believe that those things caused the abuse.

As a result, Adina decided it was not realistic or helpful to keep blaming her-self. She came up with a new alternative thought based on the evidence. Her ABC Worksheet looked like this:

A	B	C
Activating event	Belief/stuck point	Consequence
Hit in front of my daughter	I shouldn't have provoked him. It's my fault my daughter saw him hit me.	Ashamed

Are my thoughts above in B *realistic or helpful*?   <u>No, not realistic or helpful</u>

What can you tell yourself on such occasions in the future? <u>My husband is the one who</u>
<u>chose to hit me. It was not my intention, so it is not my fault.</u>

   When Adina thought about this change in thinking, she realized that her emotion changed. Whereas she was originally feeling quite ashamed, now she felt less so. She also started to notice that instead of shame, she now felt more sadness and even anger at her husband. These are actually natural emotions. They are not coming from stuck points about the event like *shoulda–coulda–wouldas* or *if onlys*. They are coming from the reality of the event, that her husband chose to hit her. Anyone would feel sad or angry thinking that their partner chose to hit them and that, by doing so, they exposed a child to something scary and hard to understand. It also makes sense to feel anger at a perpetrator. As Adina allows herself to feel these emotions, they decrease naturally over time and contribute to her recovery.

Go back over your completed ABC Worksheets about the trauma (pages 95–98) and notice if your emotions change when you tell yourself something different from the stuck point in B. Is there a decrease in the manufactured emotion in C? Do you feel any different natural emotions? If you are feeling natural emotions like sadness that the event happened or that you couldn't prevent it, allow yourself to feel those emotions. Remember that natural emotions do not last forever at the same intensity if you let yourself feel them. You don't need to do anything to stop natural emotions. Just sit there and feel them. Feeling anger doesn't mean you need to do anything. If you are still feeling emotions like guilt, shame, regret, or anger at yourself—manufactured emotions that come from the stuck point in B—you'll want to keep working to look at the evidence. Don't worry if you still believe your stuck points. You are still learning a new skill. You'll continue to work on examining the evidence for your stuck points throughout the rest of this book.

* * *

Continue tracking your PTSD Checklist symptom scores. Have you been charting your progress using the Graph for Tracking Your Weekly Scores on page 24? If not, you may wish to do so. Many people doing CPT start feeling better at this point in the program. If your symptom score is still high, don't worry. There is still plenty of time to benefit, and not everyone gets better at the same rate. Keep an eye out for avoidance and make sure that is not getting in the way of your progress.

Courtney noticed that her scores had not decreased and was discouraged at first. But after a little thought she went back to the previous two chapters to look for obstacles to her progress. She recognized that she tended not to focus on the index event. It was easier to work on everyday events. She also noticed that she wasn't completing a worksheet every day. After she went back and worked on those chapters again, she could see that her symptoms started to improve when she was focusing on the index trauma and doing worksheets more frequently.

(PTSD Checklist)

Complete the PTSD Checklist to track your symptoms as you complete this book. Be sure to complete this measure on the same index event each time. When the instructions and questions refer to a "stressful experience," remember that that is your index event—the worst event that you are working on first.

Write in here the trauma that you are working on first: _____

Complete this PTSD Checklist with reference to that event.

Instructions: Below is a list of problems that people sometimes have in response to a very stressful experience. Please read each problem carefully, and then circle one of the numbers to the right to indicate how much you have been bothered by that problem *in the past week*.

In the past week, how much were you bothered by:	Not at all	A little bit	Mod-erately	Quite a bit	Extremely
1. Repeated, disturbing, and unwanted memories of the stressful experience?	0	1	2	3	4
2. Repeated, disturbing dreams of the stressful experience?	0	1	2	3	4
3. Suddenly feeling or acting as if the stressful experience were actually happening again (*as if you were actually back there reliving it*)?	0	1	2	3	4
4. Feeling very upset when something reminded you of the stressful experience?	0	1	2	3	4
5. Having strong physical reactions when something reminded you of the stressful experience (*for example, heart pounding, trouble breathing, sweating*)?	0	1	2	3	4
6. Avoiding memories, thoughts, or feelings related to the stressful experience?	0	1	2	3	4
7. Avoiding external reminders of the stressful experience (*for example, people, places, conversations, activities, objects, or situations*)?	0	1	2	3	4
8. Trouble remembering important parts of the stressful experience (not due to head injury or substances)?	0	1	2	3	4
9. Having strong negative beliefs about yourself, other people, or the world (*for example, having thoughts such as I am bad, There is something seriously wrong with me, No one can be trusted, or The world is completely dangerous*)?	0	1	2	3	4
10. Blaming yourself or someone else (who didn't intend the outcome) for the stressful experience or what happened after it?	0	1	2	3	4
11. Having strong negative feelings, such as fear, horror, anger, guilt, or shame?	0	1	2	3	4
12. Loss of interest in activities that you used to enjoy?	0	1	2	3	4
13. Feeling distant or cut off from other people?	0	1	2	3	4
14. Trouble experiencing positive feelings (*for example, being unable to feel happiness or have loving feelings for people close to you*)?	0	1	2	3	4
15. Irritable behavior, angry outbursts, or acting aggressively?	0	1	2	3	4
16. Taking too many risks or doing things that could cause you harm?	0	1	2	3	4
17. Being "super alert" or watchful or on guard?	0	1	2	3	4
18. Feeling jumpy or easily startled?	0	1	2	3	4
19. Having difficulty concentrating?	0	1	2	3	4
20. Trouble falling or staying asleep?	0	1	2	3	4

Add up the total and write it here: _____

8

The Exploring Questions Worksheet

You're making great progress learning the first steps to get unstuck from PTSD. Keep at it, and you're likely to see a reduction in your symptoms over the next few weeks. You have already begun to examine your thoughts about why your most distressing traumatic event occurred. You've seen that what you say to yourself about the traumatic event can have a big impact on how you feel, and that when you work on the self-blame stuck points that lead to manufactured emotions, those emotions can become much less intense or change completely. Importantly, you have learned to consider the context, to decide whether the event was foreseeable and preventable, and to figure out what people and factors actually contributed to the event the most. You may have started to reconsider your ideas about your own role in the event.

This chapter teaches you how to use the Exploring Questions Worksheet on page 106. You can also download the Exploring Questions Worksheet from *www.guilford.com/resick2-forms* and make copies to fill out electronically or on paper. This worksheet can help you look even more closely at what you're saying to yourself about the trauma. It can also help you think about other situations, but at this point in CPT, be sure you are still spending some practice time each day working on your stuck points about why the traumatic event happened.

Guidance for Completing the Exploring Questions Worksheet

To complete the Exploring Questions Worksheet, you'll first pick out one of the stuck points on your log to work with, preferably one about the index traumatic event itself that leads to strong emotions. If you have any stuck points about why the event happened, such as things you "should have" done differently, or ways it could have been prevented, pick one of those and write it at the top of the worksheet where it says "Belief/stuck point." We're going to use the example "It's my fault that it happened" to help walk you through the questions. If that is a stuck point you believe, you can do a worksheet on that. If that is not one of your stuck points, choose another stuck point about why the event happened and follow

Exploring Questions Worksheet

Below is a list of questions to be used in helping you explore your stuck points. Not all questions will be appropriate for the belief/stuck point you choose to examine. Answer as many questions as you can for the belief/stuck point you have chosen to explore below.

Belief/stuck point: _____

_____

1. What is the evidence against this stuck point?

2. What information are you not including about your stuck point?

3. How does your stuck point include all-or-none terms (such as "all," "never") or extreme statements (such as "need," "should," "must," "can't," and "every time")?

4. In what way is your stuck point overfocused on just one piece of the event?

5. How is the source of information for this stuck point questionable?

6. How is your stuck point confusing something that is possible with something that is definite?

7. In what ways is your stuck point based on feelings rather than facts?

along with the instructions and examples on the next few pages to help you answer each of the questions as well as you can with regard to that stuck point. Not every question will match the stuck point you have written on the top of your worksheet, but most will. Try to answer as many of the questions as you can. Also, instead of just saying "Yes" or "No," write down enough details and specifics so that you can look back later and understand why the answer is yes or no.

Now, let's look at each question on the sheet, what they are asking, and what you might write down, using "It's my fault that it happened" as an example.

Question 1. What is the evidence against this stuck point? In other words, what information suggests it is not true? For this question, think about a court of law. What are the facts? For example, is there real factual evidence that the event is your fault, that you intentionally caused it? Consider whether there is any information that is contrary to your stuck point. Look at every word in your stuck point and also think about what your stuck point implies. For example, if you said, "It's my fault that it happened," is there a hidden or implied word in the sentence, like *all*? Is it actually *all* your fault? Is it your fault at all (did you plan and intend the outcome)? It's important to reserve the words *blame* and *fault* and therefore, the emotion *guilt* only for those events that you intended. Is there someone else who played a role or who intended the outcome? If so, it isn't all your fault (or perhaps not your fault at all). If you didn't intend the outcome, then it's time to stop using the word *fault* or *blame* automatically, as a bad habit, without thinking carefully about whether those words really apply. We all develop habits in our thinking as ways of making sense of the information that comes our way more efficiently, but sometimes these "shortcuts" leave out important information. Catch yourself every time you think that something is your fault and ask yourself if you intended a bad outcome. In this case, you might write in "I didn't intend it" or "[So-and-so] was the one who intended it" or "It was an accident. No one intended it."

Question 2. What information are you not including about your stuck point? When you think the stuck point, what are you leaving out? Sometimes when you have PTSD, you get tunnel vision. You flash back onto a single image and lose the rest of the context. You forget the role of others or don't think about what you could or couldn't have known or done at the time. For example, taking the stuck point "It's my fault that it happened," you would want to put yourself back in time and look at the full story of what happened, including all of the different factors that were at play. For example, someone who was sexually abused might blame themselves because they didn't fight back or say "No." Other details to consider that might be left out: How old were you? What were your abilities and knowledge at the time? Did you know how to prevent or stop what was happening? Did you have the physical ability to do so? How fast did the event occur, and what options did you really have? Did you perhaps even try to stop or prevent it, even if unsuccessfully? If you thought of something later that you think you could or should have done, it doesn't count. Remember that if you were having a fight, flight, or freeze reaction, it was impossible to think through every possible option clearly. Other options that might seem good in hindsight (like fighting back, or fighting harder, or not following an established protocol) might have actually led to greater harm or injury. What information are you leaving out of the story when you say the stuck point? Does this affect your assessment that it's your fault?

Question 3. How does your stuck point include all-or-none terms (such as "all," "never") or extreme statements (such as "need," "should," "must," "can't," and "every time")?

Here you are being asked to be on the lookout for words or phrases that are oversimplified or extreme. For example, if you're saying to yourself that it's *all* your fault, even if the "all" is not stated explicitly but implied, that would be an all-or-none term. If your stuck point includes words like *always, never, everyone,* or *no one,* for example, those would be all-or-none terms. Do you see how there is no in-between? It's as if there are only two options, like "Either I'm perfect or I'm a failure." In all-or-none thinking, there are no exceptions. But actually, if there is even one exception to your stuck point, it isn't true.

It's possible that the stuck point you're evaluating may not have just two categories. It might, however, have very demanding words in it like *should* or *must* that are other kinds of absolutes. For example, if you believe you "should have" been able to protect yourself from harm, that is an extreme or exaggerated way of thinking because you are leaving out the possibility that something unavoidable and that you have no control over could happen. Believing that something will "always" happen or will "never" happen may also be an extreme statement that needs to be examined more closely. Even the word *fault* is extreme or exaggerated if you did not in fact intend the outcome.

Question 4. In what way is your stuck point overfocused on just one piece of the event? This question is similar to Question 2, asking if you are taking the whole event into account. In this question, ask yourself if you are overfocusing on some small piece of the event. For example, if the stuck point was "It's my fault the assault happened because I had too much to drink," a question to ask yourself would be whether you are focusing on just your choice to drink. Were there any other factors at play? Have you or other people ever done the same thing without the outcome that happened during the traumatic event (for example, drinking without being assaulted, taking a shortcut to work without getting into a car accident, or arguing with someone without being physically threatened)? Were other people involved in the event (for example, was the drinking even relevant to the occurrence of the event, or were there other factors such as the perpetrator's intent in an assault, or the road conditions, or what other drivers were doing in a car accident that played a bigger or more important role)?

Question 5. How is the source of information for this stuck point questionable? This question is asking you to think about where you got this idea. For example, someone who had the stuck point "It's my fault that it happened" might consider that they started thinking that way after someone they told about the trauma blamed them. Or perhaps the perpetrator may have said, "You made me do it." Did you say this stuck point to yourself at the time of the trauma? Was it something you thought of later when trying to make sense of why the trauma happened? Did someone say this to you? Did you have this belief even before the traumatic event? Was it part of the just-world belief? If someone else said it was your fault, consider the source. Did they have all the facts? Might they have had some other motive (like wanting to believe that they could prevent the same thing from happening to them by doing something different)? If the person who abused you as a child told you it was your fault ("If you had behaved better, I wouldn't have had to use the belt to teach you a lesson"), are there other reasons they might want you to believe it was your fault and not theirs? Are they a balanced and unbiased source on the subject?

If you came up with the belief yourself, when and under what circumstances did you come up with the belief? Was it in the aftermath of the trauma, when distressed? Were you trying to make sense of what happened or to mentally undo it in some way? Were you young enough that you made sense of what happened through the just-world belief because you weren't able to identify all of the more complex factors at play in what happened? Remember that the just-world belief is when people say that if something bad happens to someone, it's because they weren't careful enough or did something "wrong." Consider whether the just-world belief is a one hundred percent true, reliable source of information on this stuck point. Is the just-world belief always true? If there are ever times it isn't true, it's a questionable source. Or consider, is the belief coming from you in hindsight? Remember that hindsight is not a dependable source because it's based on what you know now, not what you knew then. Did you consider the idea carefully, taking into consideration all of the facts, or was it based more on emotions? If the stuck point is not based on the facts, then it's a questionable source. That doesn't mean you are a questionable person or source—it just means that the circumstances that led to that particular belief might have been questionable (if you were emotionally distressed, just trying to make sense of it, came up with it when you were much younger, etc.).

Question 6. How is your stuck point confusing something that is possible with something that is definite? This question is often helpful when you feel anxious or fearful of potential future events. It asks you to consider whether you are taking something that is "possible" and assuming that it is "likely" to occur—for example, if you say, "If I go to the shopping mall, there *will* be a shooting." It's possible that something like that will happen, but is it actually definite? Would you bet all of your savings on the idea that something will definitely happen? Maybe not if the chances are small and it's only possible, not likely.

If you blame yourself for what happened, you can also ask yourself how likely it is that it is all your fault. You can ask yourself how probable it is that any stuck point is true.

Question 7. In what ways is your stuck point based on feelings rather than facts? For example, if something terrible happens to you and you started to feel guilty or ashamed, you might start to think that you must have done something wrong. In other words, you think backward from how you feel as proof of a thought. Another example would be feeling fear and assuming that you must be in danger. Notice if your stuck point is based on facts or more based on emotions. If it is based on emotions, which emotions are you basing your thoughts on?

On pages 110–111 you will find two completed examples of the Exploring Questions Worksheet. Notice that the responses are somewhat detailed. This approach is helpful because if you take the time to really think through each question, the worksheets can be something you can look back on later if you notice that you are still thinking the stuck point out of habit. Answering the questions may help you reevaluate your stuck points, and you may change your thinking. It's also normal to go through this process and start to believe

Example Exploring Questions Worksheet

Belief/stuck point: _It's command's fault my friend was killed because they didn't do a thorough risk assessment before sending us to that position. (Combat)_

1. What is the evidence against this stuck point?

   They didn't intend for us to be hit.

2. What information are you not including about your stuck point?

   It doesn't include the enemy that shot the rocket.

3. How does your stuck point include all-or-none terms (such as "all," "never") or extreme statements (such as "need," "should," "must," "can't," and "every time")?

   It's suggesting it's all their fault. Even if they were negligent, they didn't intend for it to happen.

4. In what way is your stuck point over-focused on just one piece of the story?

   I'm focusing on the risk assessment and that it wasn't done for this mission. I guess what I'm not taking into account is that there have been casualties on other missions even if a risk assessment was done. Casualties are part of war.

5. How is the source of information for this stuck point questionable?

   It came from me and some of the other guys in my unit. We were really angry that our buddy was killed and wanted somewhere to direct the anger.

6. How is your stuck point confusing something that is possible with something that is definite?

   It's possible that a risk assessment might have led to a change in the plan, but not necessarily.

7. In what ways is your stuck point based on feelings rather than facts?

   It's based on feelings—I feel angry, and this leads me to point to leadership.

the stuck point less, but still believe it a little bit. Continuing to read over your answers can help you "chip away" when you still have the habit of thinking the stuck point or if you still feel the emotions that arise from the stuck point.

> ▶▶ To watch a video to review what you just read here about using the Exploring Questions Worksheet, go to the CPT Whiteboard Video Library (*http://cptforptsd.com/cpt-resources*) and watch the video called *How to Fill Out an Exploring Questions Worksheet*. You can also watch a video called *Exploring Questions Worksheet Example*.

Example Exploring Questions Worksheet

Belief/stuck point: I should have evacuated sooner. (Natural disaster)

_____

1. What is the evidence against this stuck point?

   I didn't know the hurricane would hit so fast or hard.

2. What information are you not including about your stuck point?

   There have been other hurricane warnings in our area before, but none were this bad.

3. How does your stuck point include all-or-none terms (such as "all," "never") or extreme statements (such as "need," "should," "must," "can't," and "every time")?

   It includes a "should" and implies that I didn't try to evacuate at all. I did eventually, but it was too late by then.

4. In what way is your stuck point over-focused on just one piece of the story?

   I am focusing on my delaying evacuating, but not that I did try to leave and also helped other people stay safe.

5. How is the source of information for this stuck point questionable?

   It comes from me but also people on TV saying it's people's own fault if they don't evacuate when they're told. They don't really know what it's like and how hard it is to leave your home. I also didn't really have an obvious place to go while some people might have had family or friends who could take them in.

6. How is your stuck point confusing something that is possible with something that is definite?

   It's possible but not likely I would have known how bad things would get so quickly.

7. In what ways is your stuck point based on feelings rather than facts?

   It's definitely based on feelings of guilt and embarrassment.

PRACTICE ASSIGNMENT

Complete at least one Exploring Questions Worksheet (see pages 113–117) per day over the next week with regard to your stuck points about the trauma. Continue to prioritize stuck points about why the trauma happened, such as your stuck points about blame, _shoulda–coulda–wouldas,_ and _if onlys._ Write the stuck point at the top of the page and keep referring back to it as you answer the questions. Remember, you are not evaluating the traumatic event but your thoughts about why it happened. Refer back to the instructions and to the examples of completed Exploring Questions Worksheets to help you.

It's worth mentioning that many people find the Exploring Questions Worksheet a bit daunting at first. However, just do your best and don't worry if you're doing it "perfectly." Watch the videos mentioned on page 110 for some help. But do keep practicing at least a little bit every day. This part of the program is when people start seeing changes in their thinking and symptoms, so don't give up now! Keep up the work you've been putting in and refer back to your goals and reasons you are doing this if you need to.

 ## TROUBLESHOOTING

What if I don't understand all the questions on the worksheet?

That's OK! The Exploring Questions Worksheet is simply a tool to help you evaluate what you have been saying to yourself. Some of the questions may make more sense with some stuck points than others. If you don't know what to write in response to one of the questions, you can skip it and move on to the next. But don't give up on doing the worksheet because one of the questions doesn't make sense or apply to a particular stuck point. The next question might be just the one you need to reconsider the event in an important way.

My answers to some of the questions are the same as to previous questions.

It's possible that your answers will be the same or redundant, and that's OK. There are slight differences between some of the questions because different wording may make more sense with different stuck points or click more for you than others. Again, if you're not sure what a question is asking, go back and look at the explanations to see what the differences between questions are.

I can't answer all of the questions on my stuck point. What if a question doesn't make sense for my stuck point?

It's fine if you don't answer every question, but try to do so when you can. Not every question fits every stuck point. That's why we have seven different questions you can use to examine your thoughts.

*   *   *

After you complete some Exploring Questions Worksheets, turn to page 118 (or *www. guilford.com/resick2-forms*) and complete another PTSD checklist to see if your symptoms are changing. How are your symptoms changing over time? Are you noticing any change from week to week on the Graph for Tracking Your Weekly Scores found on page 24? In which symptoms are you noticing change? In which areas are you still experiencing the most symptoms?

Exploring Questions Worksheet

Below is a list of questions to be used in helping you explore your stuck points. Not all questions will be appropriate for the belief/stuck point you choose to examine. Answer as many questions as you can for the belief/stuck point you have chosen to explore below.

Belief/stuck point: _____

_____

1. What is the evidence against this stuck point?

2. What information are you not including about your stuck point?

3. How does your stuck point include all-or-none terms (such as "all," "never") or extreme statements (such as "need," "should," "must," "can't," and "every time")?

4. In what way is your stuck point overfocused on just one piece of the event?

5. How is the source of information for this stuck point questionable?

6. How is your stuck point confusing something that is possible with something that is definite?

7. In what ways is your stuck point based on feelings rather than facts?

Exploring Questions Worksheet

Below is a list of questions to be used in helping you explore your stuck points. Not all questions will be appropriate for the belief/stuck point you choose to examine. Answer as many questions as you can for the belief/stuck point you have chosen to explore below.

Belief/stuck point: _____

_____

1. What is the evidence against this stuck point?

2. What information are you not including about your stuck point?

3. How does your stuck point include all-or-none terms (such as "all," "never") or extreme statements (such as "need," "should," "must," "can't," and "every time")?

4. In what way is your stuck point overfocused on just one piece of the event?

5. How is the source of information for this stuck point questionable?

6. How is your stuck point confusing something that is possible with something that is definite?

7. In what ways is your stuck point based on feelings rather than facts?

Exploring Questions Worksheet

Below is a list of questions to be used in helping you explore your stuck points. Not all questions will be appropriate for the belief/stuck point you choose to examine. Answer as many questions as you can for the belief/stuck point you have chosen to explore below.

Belief/stuck point: _____

_____

1. What is the evidence against this stuck point?

2. What information are you not including about your stuck point?

3. How does your stuck point include all-or-none terms (such as "all," "never") or extreme statements (such as "need," "should," "must," "can't," and "every time")?

4. In what way is your stuck point overfocused on just one piece of the event?

5. How is the source of information for this stuck point questionable?

6. How is your stuck point confusing something that is possible with something that is definite?

7. In what ways is your stuck point based on feelings rather than facts?

Exploring Questions Worksheet

Below is a list of questions to be used in helping you explore your stuck points. Not all questions will be appropriate for the belief/stuck point you choose to examine. Answer as many questions as you can for the belief/stuck point you have chosen to explore below.

Belief/stuck point: _____

_____

1. What is the evidence against this stuck point?

2. What information are you not including about your stuck point?

3. How does your stuck point include all-or-none terms (such as "all," "never") or extreme statements (such as "need," "should," "must," "can't," and "every time")?

4. In what way is your stuck point overfocused on just one piece of the event?

5. How is the source of information for this stuck point questionable?

6. How is your stuck point confusing something that is possible with something that is definite?

7. In what ways is your stuck point based on feelings rather than facts?

Exploring Questions Worksheet

Below is a list of questions to be used in helping you explore your stuck points. Not all questions will be appropriate for the belief/stuck point you choose to examine. Answer as many questions as you can for the belief/stuck point you have chosen to explore below.

Belief/stuck point: _____

_____

1. What is the evidence against this stuck point?

2. What information are you not including about your stuck point?

3. How does your stuck point include all-or-none terms (such as "all," "never") or extreme statements (such as "need," "should," "must," "can't," and "every time")?

4. In what way is your stuck point overfocused on just one piece of the event?

5. How is the source of information for this stuck point questionable?

6. How is your stuck point confusing something that is possible with something that is definite?

7. In what ways is your stuck point based on feelings rather than facts?

⟨PTSD Checklist⟩

Complete the PTSD Checklist to track your symptoms as you complete this book. Be sure to complete this measure on the same index event each time. When the instructions and questions refer to a "stressful experience," remember that that is your index event—the worst event that you are working on first.

Write in here the trauma that you are working on first: _____

Complete this PTSD Checklist with reference to that event.

Instructions: Below is a list of problems that people sometimes have in response to a very stressful experience. Please read each problem carefully, and then circle one of the numbers to the right to indicate how much you have been bothered by that problem *in the past week*.

In the past week, how much were you bothered by:	Not at all	A little bit	Moderately	Quite a bit	Extremely
1. Repeated, disturbing, and unwanted memories of the stressful experience?	0	1	2	3	4
2. Repeated, disturbing dreams of the stressful experience?	0	1	2	3	4
3. Suddenly feeling or acting as if the stressful experience were actually happening again (*as if you were actually back there reliving it*)?	0	1	2	3	4
4. Feeling very upset when something reminded you of the stressful experience?	0	1	2	3	4
5. Having strong physical reactions when something reminded you of the stressful experience (*for example, heart pounding, trouble breathing, sweating*)?	0	1	2	3	4
6. Avoiding memories, thoughts, or feelings related to the stressful experience?	0	1	2	3	4
7. Avoiding external reminders of the stressful experience (*for example, people, places, conversations, activities, objects, or situations*)?	0	1	2	3	4
8. Trouble remembering important parts of the stressful experience (not due to head injury or substances)?	0	1	2	3	4
9. Having strong negative beliefs about yourself, other people, or the world (*for example, having thoughts such as I am bad, There is something seriously wrong with me, No one can be trusted, or The world is completely dangerous*)?	0	1	2	3	4
10. Blaming yourself or someone else (who didn't intend the outcome) for the stressful experience or what happened after it?	0	1	2	3	4
11. Having strong negative feelings, such as fear, horror, anger, guilt, or shame?	0	1	2	3	4
12. Loss of interest in activities that you used to enjoy?	0	1	2	3	4
13. Feeling distant or cut off from other people?	0	1	2	3	4
14. Trouble experiencing positive feelings (*for example, being unable to feel happiness or have loving feelings for people close to you*)?	0	1	2	3	4
15. Irritable behavior, angry outbursts, or acting aggressively?	0	1	2	3	4
16. Taking too many risks or doing things that could cause you harm?	0	1	2	3	4
17. Being "super alert" or watchful or on guard?	0	1	2	3	4
18. Feeling jumpy or easily startled?	0	1	2	3	4
19. Having difficulty concentrating?	0	1	2	3	4
20. Trouble falling or staying asleep?	0	1	2	3	4

Add up the total and write it here: _____

From *PTSD Checklist for DSM-5 (PCL-5)* by Weathers, Litz, Keane, Palmieri, Marx, and Schnurr (2013). Available from the National Center for PTSD at *www.ptsd.va.gov*; in the public domain. Reprinted in *Getting Unstuck from PTSD* (Guilford Press, 2023). Purchasers of this book can photocopy and/or download additional copies of this worksheet at *www.guilford.com/resick2-forms* for personal use or use with clients; see copyright page for details.

9

Introducing Thinking Patterns

How did it go with the Exploring Questions Worksheets? Were you able to use the questions to identify any new, helpful ways of looking at your trauma? If so, give yourself some praise. Don't worry if you didn't understand every question perfectly or haven't changed your way of thinking yet. You are continuing to build a set of skills to examine your thoughts, and you will have more opportunities to continue to benefit with the next set of skills. Now that you have been practicing examining the facts about one stuck point at a time, you can use this chapter to see if you have patterns of thinking that are unhelpful to you and keep you stuck in your PTSD.

A key thing to remember is that everyone develops patterns in their thinking—they can be helpful shortcuts as we have learned to categorize and organize information that comes our way every day. People pick up habits in their thinking as ways of taking in information and processing it more efficiently. These patterns are habitual ways of thinking that occur not just when you think about your traumatic events but when everyday events occur as well.

However, for people with PTSD and other problems like depression and anxiety, some of these patterns come too easily and lead to a lot of negative conclusions. They might become habits that are no longer helpful. Maybe you've been relying on these patterns in your thinking too much and they're no longer leading you to the most balanced or helpful conclusions. Some patterns can also keep people from interacting with the world and get in the way of healthy relationships.

In this chapter, you'll first identify whether any of your stuck points are examples of common **thinking patterns**. After you've identified which patterns some of your stuck points fall into, you can begin to catch yourself when you find yourself using them in your everyday life as well and complete the Thinking Patterns Worksheets found on pages 125–131. You can also download and print the worksheet from *www.guilford.com/resick2-forms*. For example, if you find yourself thinking "I bet this person wants to take advantage of me" when you interact with someone new, you can remind yourself that you might be jumping to conclusions or mind reading and that you don't know enough about them to know what their intentions are. This can help you slow down and think through a situation before you make a snap judgment about what to do.

As you read about the patterns below, you may notice some overlap between the patterns and the questions you were asking yourself in the last chapter. Being able to recognize and name the pattern helps some people slow down and ask themselves questions about what they're saying to themselves or how they're reacting to situations that trigger their stuck points.

You may have just some of these tendencies, or you may discover examples of all of them in your stuck points. Some of the common patterns are the following:

1. Jumping to conclusions or predicting the future. We all want to feel a sense of control over the things that happen to us and want to believe that we can anticipate what will happen. Sometimes we have a tendency to make assumptions without checking the facts or think that we know what will happen in the future. For example, if you were hurt by others in the past, you may assume "If I trust someone, they will hurt me." Anytime you declare what "will" happen in the future or make a connection between two things that may or may not be connected, you are jumping to conclusions.

Look over your Stuck Point Log (page 56). Do you see any examples of jumping to conclusions in it? Write down an example here:

_____

_____

_____

_____

2. Ignoring important parts of a situation—what are you leaving out? Sometimes when people think about why an event happened, they forget to take into account the entire context of the situation. For example, looking back at your index trauma, are you ignoring factors like:

- How young you were when it happened
- What you actually knew at the time going into the situation
- How much time you had to figure out what was going on and what to do
- Who had the intent for the outcome
- Who else was there and what roles they played

An example is someone believing they should have fought back and stopped abuse that happened when they were a small child. They are ignoring the fact that they were much younger, smaller, frightened, and didn't have the ability to actually fight off someone who was much bigger than they were. If you thought of something later that you might have tried to stop the event but you didn't think of that or weren't able to do that at the time, then it doesn't count. Another way that people ignore important parts of a situation are to focus only on their "failures" and not their successes. Sometimes in a dangerous situation people successfully act in ways that help to preserve their lives or their health, or those of others, but they forget to acknowledge that later and focus only on not having stopped the event altogether. For example, an emergency responder might focus on the person who they could not save instead of on the others that they did help.

Look over your Stuck Point Log. Do you see any examples of ignoring important parts of a situation? Write down an example here:

_____

_____

_____

_____

3. Oversimplifying things as good–bad or right–wrong or "**overgeneralizing**" from a single incident (for example, applying one experience too broadly). Sometimes people have only two categories for things, especially if the traumatic event occurred when they were young and they had not yet learned that most things fall on a continuum. For example, they may label someone as "untrustworthy" if they make a single mistake and ignore all the other good or neutral things they have done. You might find yourself being overly judgmental of others or yourself. For example, if you say to yourself, "If I'm not perfect, then I'm a failure," you're using only two categories in your grading system. What would you think of a teacher who said, "A 100% correct is an A and a 99% is an F"? If you're being perfectionistic, your grading system is unreasonably strict. Look at your Stuck Point Log and notice how many statements include or imply just two categories. Do you do this with people and events generally? Is this one of your tendencies?

Similarly, overgeneralizing is a tendency to assume that if one bad thing happens, it will always happen. Again, you are not taking into account all of the exceptions, all of the neutral days or good days, and you might be assuming that if you have had a traumatic event occur to you, it **will** happen again. Or you might assume that it is never safe to go out at night or to go to certain places when, in fact, most of the time nothing bad would happen in that situation. Overgeneralizing is assuming something is "always" the case or thinking that "everyone" fits a certain category.

Look over your Stuck Point Log. Do you see any examples of oversimplifying or over-generalizing? Write down an example here:

_____

_____

_____

_____

4. Mind reading (assuming that people are thinking negatively of you or have negative intentions when there is no definite evidence for this). This common pattern of thinking involves believing that people are thinking negatively about you or that they think the same as you do. Instead of asking why someone did something, you may make assumptions about how they must be thinking or what their reasons are. Often we assume others have negative thoughts or intentions. Some examples are "They don't want to spend time with me" or "They're trying to make me angry." Many people wonder if other people can tell that they have experienced trauma and are judging them for it. Others assume that other people have bad intentions or ulterior motives. Anytime you assume what someone else is thinking, feeling, or intending without their telling you, it's mind reading.

Look over your Stuck Point Log. Do you see any examples of mind reading? Write down an example here:

_____

_____

_____

_____

5. **Emotional reasoning** (using your emotions as proof of your stuck point). This is the tendency to start from how you feel and then use that as proof that your stuck point must be correct. When someone is triggered by a trauma reminder, it's common to feel fear or panic and believe something like "I feel fear, so I must be in danger." Because trauma can lead people's alarm systems to be very sensitive, and you may experience many false alarms, be careful about assuming you are always actually in danger. Fear doesn't always indicate danger. Another common example is "Because I feel guilty, I must have done something wrong." Emotions are the outcome of events or thoughts, but they aren't reliable as the reason to think a thought. You cannot use your emotions as proof of your stuck points because if you change your thoughts, your emotions will change. When you experience emotional reasoning, you may notice that it's a habit of thinking, not a fact.

Look over your Stuck Point Log. Do you see any examples of emotional reasoning? Write down an example here:

_____

_____

_____

_____

Now that you've learned the common thinking patterns, complete some of the Thinking Patterns Worksheets provided on pages 125–131 to continue to practice noticing examples of the patterns in your stuck points and in your everyday thoughts. You can also download the Thinking Patterns Worksheets from *www.guilford.com/resick2-forms* and make copies to fill out electronically or on paper. Also refer to the filled-in example worksheets on pages 123 and 124.

As with the Exploring Questions Worksheets examples, notice that the responses are somewhat detailed. If you take the time to really think through how your stuck points fall into the different patterns, you can start to catch yourself when you think one of your stuck points, notice that it is one of the thinking patterns, and remind yourself to think it through instead of falling automatically into the pattern.

Example Thinking Patterns Worksheet

1. **Jumping to conclusions** or **predicting the future.**

   If I speak up, no one will listen to me—I'm assuming no one will listen because I wasn't believed when I spoke up about the military sexual trauma, but I don't know that other people will be the same. I have sometimes spoken up at work and my boss listened.

2. **Ignoring important parts** of a situation.

   I let it happen—this is ignoring that I tried fighting back at first. After that I just wanted it to be over with as fast as possible.

3. **Oversimplifying** things as "good—bad" or "right—wrong" or **overgeneralizing** from a single incident (applying one experience too broadly).

   No one can be trusted—it's overgeneralizing to say "no one" can be trusted just because some people couldn't be. I have known some people who were trustworthy.

4. **Mind reading** (assuming that people are thinking negatively of you when there is no definite evidence for this).

   No one will want me now—this assumes what other people will think and feel about my past. They may not really feel this way.

5. **Emotional reasoning** (using your emotions as proof—for example, "I feel fear, so I must be in danger").

   Men are not safe to be alone with—I feel uncomfortable around men since I was raped, so I assume I am in danger. But I have been alone with men before without being assaulted.

> ▶▶ To watch a video to review what you just read about the Thinking Patterns Worksheet, go to the CPT Whiteboard Video Library (*http://cptforptsd.com/cpt-resources*) and watch the video called *How to Fill Out a Thinking Patterns Worksheet*. You can also watch a video called *Thinking Patterns Worksheet Example*.

 PRACTICE ASSIGNMENT

Complete a Thinking Patterns Worksheet every day for the next week (see pages 125–131), noticing patterns from your everyday life as well as in your thinking about your traumatic events. Refer to your Stuck Point Log and categorize each stuck point to see if it falls into any of the patterns. Also notice your everyday thoughts and see if any of these fit under any of the patterns. For example, if someone cancels plans with you, notice whether you mind read what the reason was for canceling ("They don't want to see me").

Keep in mind that a stuck point could fit into more than one category. Also keep in mind that there might be hidden words in your stuck point. For example, when you say that people are untrustworthy, are you really thinking "all" people are untrustworthy? That stuck point might fit under jumping to conclusions, ignoring important parts of a situation, or oversimplifying/overgeneralizing. So there is not one right answer. You're just practicing the skill of noticing whether any of your thoughts fall into any of the patterns so you can become more adept at noticing it when it's happening.

After you have done several Thinking Patterns Worksheets, or worked on this each day for a week, look across all of the Thinking Patterns Worksheets that you completed before moving on to the next chapter. Do you notice whether you are engaging in many or all of the patterns? Or do you "specialize" in one or two of the patterns in particular (for example, mind reading or jumping to conclusions)? What do you notice about your patterns, with regard to both your trauma and everyday situations?

_____

_____

_____

_____

Example Thinking Patterns Worksheet

1. **Jumping to conclusions** or **predicting the future.**

   I'm going to become like my parents—assuming that because I witnessed their violence I will succumb to the same fate. But I have had positive relationships without abuse.

2. **Ignoring important parts** of a situation.

   I should have been able to stop them—this ignores that I did try to stop it, sometimes calling 911, but I didn't really have control over them. Also I was just a kid, and it was not really my responsibility to stop grown adults from trying to hurt each other.

3. **Oversimplifying** things as "good—bad" or "right—wrong" or **overgeneralizing** from a single incident (applying one experience too broadly).

   Intimacy is dangerous—I assume because of my childhood that anytime a couple gets close they are likely to become violent, but that is not always the case.

4. **Mind reading** (assuming that people are thinking negatively of you when there is no definite evidence for this).

   No one will ever understand me—I assume no one can understand me, but other people may have also been through trauma like me and have an idea of what it's like.

5. **Emotional reasoning** (using your emotions as proof—for example, "I feel fear, so I must be in danger").

   I am damaged—I feel sad and scared sometimes and assume this means there is something wrong with me.

Thinking Patterns Worksheet

Listed below are several different patterns of thinking that people use in different life situations. These patterns often become automatic, habitual thoughts that cause us to engage in self-defeating behavior. Considering your own stuck points, or samples from your everyday thinking, find examples for each of these patterns. Write in the stuck point or typical thought under the appropriate pattern and describe how it fits that pattern. Think about how that pattern affects you.

1. **Jumping to conclusions** or **predicting the future.**

2. **Ignoring important parts** of a situation.

3. **Oversimplifying** things as "good—bad" or "right—wrong" or **overgeneralizing** from a single incident (applying one experience too broadly).

4. **Mind reading** (assuming that people are thinking negatively of you when there is no definite evidence for this).

5. **Emotional reasoning** (using your emotions as proof—for example, "I feel fear, so I must be in danger").

Thinking Patterns Worksheet

Listed below are several different patterns of thinking that people use in different life situations. These patterns often become automatic, habitual thoughts that cause us to engage in self-defeating behavior. Considering your own stuck points, or samples from your everyday thinking, find examples for each of these patterns. Write in the stuck point or typical thought under the appropriate pattern and describe how it fits that pattern. Think about how that pattern affects you.

1. **Jumping to conclusions** or **predicting the future.**

2. **Ignoring important parts** of a situation.

3. **Oversimplifying** things as "good—bad" or "right—wrong" or **overgeneralizing** from a single incident (applying one experience too broadly).

4. **Mind reading** (assuming that people are thinking negatively of you when there is no definite evidence for this).

5. **Emotional reasoning** (using your emotions as proof—for example, "I feel fear, so I must be in danger").

Thinking Patterns Worksheet

Listed below are several different patterns of thinking that people use in different life situations. These patterns often become automatic, habitual thoughts that cause us to engage in self-defeating behavior. Considering your own stuck points, or samples from your everyday thinking, find examples for each of these patterns. Write in the stuck point or typical thought under the appropriate pattern and describe how it fits that pattern. Think about how that pattern affects you.

1. **Jumping to conclusions** or **predicting the future.**

2. **Ignoring important parts** of a situation.

3. **Oversimplifying** things as "good—bad" or "right—wrong" or **overgeneralizing** from a single incident (applying one experience too broadly).

4. **Mind reading** (assuming that people are thinking negatively of you when there is no definite evidence for this).

5. **Emotional reasoning** (using your emotions as proof—for example, "I feel fear, so I must be in danger").

Thinking Patterns Worksheet

Listed below are several different patterns of thinking that people use in different life situations. These patterns often become automatic, habitual thoughts that cause us to engage in self-defeating behavior. Considering your own stuck points, or samples from your everyday thinking, find examples for each of these patterns. Write in the stuck point or typical thought under the appropriate pattern and describe how it fits that pattern. Think about how that pattern affects you.

1. **Jumping to conclusions** or **predicting the future.**

2. **Ignoring important parts** of a situation.

3. **Oversimplifying** things as "good—bad" or "right—wrong" or **overgeneralizing** from a single incident (applying one experience too broadly).

4. **Mind reading** (assuming that people are thinking negatively of you when there is no definite evidence for this).

5. **Emotional reasoning** (using your emotions as proof—for example, "I feel fear, so I must be in danger").

Thinking Patterns Worksheet

Listed below are several different patterns of thinking that people use in different life situations. These patterns often become automatic, habitual thoughts that cause us to engage in self-defeating behavior. Considering your own stuck points, or samples from your everyday thinking, find examples for each of these patterns. Write in the stuck point or typical thought under the appropriate pattern and describe how it fits that pattern. Think about how that pattern affects you.

1. **Jumping to conclusions** or **predicting the future.**

2. **Ignoring important parts** of a situation.

3. **Oversimplifying** things as "good—bad" or "right—wrong" or **overgeneralizing** from a single incident (applying one experience too broadly).

4. **Mind reading** (assuming that people are thinking negatively of you when there is no definite evidence for this).

5. **Emotional reasoning** (using your emotions as proof—for example, "I feel fear, so I must be in danger").

Thinking Patterns Worksheet

Listed below are several different patterns of thinking that people use in different life situations. These patterns often become automatic, habitual thoughts that cause us to engage in self-defeating behavior. Considering your own stuck points, or samples from your everyday thinking, find examples for each of these patterns. Write in the stuck point or typical thought under the appropriate pattern and describe how it fits that pattern. Think about how that pattern affects you.

1. **Jumping to conclusions** or **predicting the future.**

2. **Ignoring important parts** of a situation.

3. **Oversimplifying** things as "good—bad" or "right—wrong" or **overgeneralizing** from a single incident (applying one experience too broadly).

4. **Mind reading** (assuming that people are thinking negatively of you when there is no definite evidence for this).

5. **Emotional reasoning** (using your emotions as proof—for example, "I feel fear, so I must be in danger").

Listed below are several different patterns of thinking that people use in different life situations. These patterns often become automatic, habitual thoughts that cause us to engage in self-defeating behavior. Considering your own stuck points, or samples from your everyday thinking, find examples for each of these patterns. Write in the stuck point or typical thought under the appropriate pattern and describe how it fits that pattern. Think about how that pattern affects you.

1. **Jumping to conclusions** or **predicting the future.**

2. **Ignoring important parts** of a situation.

3. **Oversimplifying** things as "good—bad" or "right—wrong" or **overgeneralizing** from a single incident (applying one experience too broadly).

4. **Mind reading** (assuming that people are thinking negatively of you when there is no definite evidence for this).

5. **Emotional reasoning** (using your emotions as proof—for example, "I feel fear, so I must be in danger").

How do you think these thinking patterns might have influenced the way you made sense of your trauma? For example, if you have noticed that you sometimes jump to conclusions, could that have contributed to your blaming yourself for the event?

_____

_____

_____

_____

If you have a pattern of thinking that has become a habit, it will be important to notice when you use it, for everyday events as well as for the trauma. These kinds of patterns can lead you to think in ways that are not helpful, are too extreme, and leave you feeling bad about yourself or others. These patterns are habits, and that means it takes practice to change these automatic ways of thinking.

It's also important to reflect on how these patterns play out in your life. Do they keep you from forming deeper relationships or from meeting goals in your life? Do they lead to conflict with others? Do they keep you isolated or feeling bad about yourself? What have you noticed about the impact of these patterns on how you live your day-to-day life?

_____

_____

_____

_____

What have you noticed about how these patterns impact your relationships with others?

_____

_____

_____

_____

When you notice these patterns coming up, it's a good sign that you could benefit from stopping and completing a worksheet to examine the stuck point more closely.

After several days of completing the Thinking Patterns Worksheets, Chris noticed that her mother tended to jump to conclusions frequently. She suddenly realized that was where she had picked up that habit. Many of her stuck points fell under the category of jumping to conclusions. She made a lot of predictions about the future, like "People will judge me," "Something bad will happen," and "I will make a bad decision." She also noticed that she tended to use emotional reasoning a great deal.

She assumed because she felt guilt as an automatic response (probably due to jumping to conclusions), that she must have done something wrong. She never stopped long enough to decide if she had in fact done something wrong or made a mistake. She just used her guilt as proof of her stuck point. Once she noticed this vicious circle between jumping to conclusions and guilt, she was able to catch herself more in the moment.

 TROUBLESHOOTING

Is it bad that I have many or all of the patterns of thinking?

No, it is not bad if you find examples of all of them. Many people with and without PTSD have these common patterns of thinking. They become more troublesome when you do have PTSD because you tend to think about the traumatic events and your future through the lens of these patterns. It's actually good that you notice them now because if you become aware of them, you can start to examine whether the conclusions you come up with are completely accurate instead of just assuming they are true. Each time you notice one, it's a cue to slow down and reconsider what you're saying to yourself.

What am I supposed to do about these patterns?

Notice when you slide into one of these patterns so that you can catch and correct yourself. They are habits that can change with practice. The next worksheet, the Alternative Thoughts Worksheet, will bring all of these concepts together and you'll get lots of practice. The important takeaway in this chapter is to understand how they are helping keep you stuck in your PTSD. The faster you learn to recognize them and adjust your thoughts, the sooner you'll recover from your PTSD. Often at this point in the process people start recognizing and correcting the subtle extremes in their stuck points, like recognizing that they are not in danger "everywhere, all the time" or that it's not true that if they make a decision, it "never" works out. Just a simple change from "everyone" to "some people" or "always" to "sometimes" can have a big impact on how you feel and how you live your life.

I'm not sure I'm putting my thought in the right category.

A single stuck point could fit into more than one category, so there is no one "right" category. For example, a stuck point like "It's all my fault that it happened" could be an example of ignoring important parts of the situation, jumping to conclusions, oversimplifying, and emotional reasoning. You might try to figure out if one is a stronger type of thinking for you. Do you tend more to jump to conclusions, engage in emotional reasoning, or something else? *Don't worry about "getting it right."* Just noticing that your stuck points are part of a pattern of thinking is enough to help you slow down and start examining the stuck points more closely.

I feel bad that I have these patterns. It's so stupid of me to think this way.

These patterns come up for people with and without PTSD. It's a way to organize information and try to have a sense of control. The things you say to yourself when you're judging yourself for having the patterns are stuck points. Take a close look at them and don't beat yourself up for taking the same mental shortcuts that everyone else does. Just use the patterns as information that it's a good time to take a look at what you're saying to yourself. When you notice a stuck point or pattern, slow down and examine the stuck points as you work on your worksheets for practice. When you start changing your thinking, it's not helpful to beat yourself up for having thought differently before. You are learning something new!

*   *   *

After you have done the worksheets for a few days, it's time to check your progress again with the PTSD Checklist. How are your symptoms coming along? Are you noticing any reductions yet looking at your scores from week to week or on your Graph for Tracking Your Weekly Scores on page 24? The next worksheet in Chapter 10 will help you put together everything you have been learning and may help you lower your symptoms even more.

(PTSD Checklist)

Complete the PTSD Checklist to track your symptoms as you complete this book. Be sure to complete this measure on the same index event each time. When the instructions and questions refer to a "stressful experience," remember that that is your index event—the worst event that you are working on first.

Write in here the trauma that you are working on first: _____

Complete this PTSD Checklist with reference to that event.

Instructions: Below is a list of problems that people sometimes have in response to a very stressful experience. Please read each problem carefully, and then circle one of the numbers to the right to indicate how much you have been bothered by that problem *in the past week*.

In the past week, how much were you bothered by:	Not at all	A little bit	Mod- erately	Quite a bit	Extremely
1. Repeated, disturbing, and unwanted memories of the stressful experience?	0	1	2	3	4
2. Repeated, disturbing dreams of the stressful experience?	0	1	2	3	4
3. Suddenly feeling or acting as if the stressful experience were actually happening again (*as if you were actually back there reliving it*)?	0	1	2	3	4
4. Feeling very upset when something reminded you of the stressful experience?	0	1	2	3	4
5. Having strong physical reactions when something reminded you of the stressful experience (*for example, heart pounding, trouble breathing, sweating*)?	0	1	2	3	4
6. Avoiding memories, thoughts, or feelings related to the stressful experience?	0	1	2	3	4
7. Avoiding external reminders of the stressful experience (*for example, people, places, conversations, activities, objects, or situations*)?	0	1	2	3	4
8. Trouble remembering important parts of the stressful experience (not due to head injury or substances)?	0	1	2	3	4
9. Having strong negative beliefs about yourself, other people, or the world (*for example, having thoughts such as I am bad, There is something seriously wrong with me, No one can be trusted, or The world is completely dangerous*)?	0	1	2	3	4
10. Blaming yourself or someone else (who didn't intend the outcome) for the stressful experience or what happened after it?	0	1	2	3	4
11. Having strong negative feelings, such as fear, horror, anger, guilt, or shame?	0	1	2	3	4
12. Loss of interest in activities that you used to enjoy?	0	1	2	3	4
13. Feeling distant or cut off from other people?	0	1	2	3	4
14. Trouble experiencing positive feelings (*for example, being unable to feel happiness or have loving feelings for people close to you*)?	0	1	2	3	4
15. Irritable behavior, angry outbursts, or acting aggressively?	0	1	2	3	4
16. Taking too many risks or doing things that could cause you harm?	0	1	2	3	4
17. Being "super alert" or watchful or on guard?	0	1	2	3	4
18. Feeling jumpy or easily startled?	0	1	2	3	4
19. Having difficulty concentrating?	0	1	2	3	4
20. Trouble falling or staying asleep?	0	1	2	3	4

Add up the total and write it here: _____

10

Using the Alternative Thoughts Worksheet to Balance Your Thinking

You have now learned several processes for examining your stuck points: first labeling them and understanding what emotions they bring up (ABC Worksheets, pages 95–98), then examining them by asking questions (Exploring Questions Worksheets, pages 113–117), and finally identifying the thinking patterns that they fall under (Thinking Patterns Worksheets, pages 125–131). Now you're ready to put the whole process together and identify things you might want to say to yourself instead that may be more balanced and realistic.

~~~~~~~~~~ Instructions for Completing ~~~~~~~~~~
the Alternative Thoughts Worksheet

The next worksheet is the final worksheet to be introduced: the Alternative Thoughts Worksheet. You'll use the Alternative Thoughts Worksheets throughout the rest of your work as you continue to consider your stuck points.

Take a look at the Alternative Thoughts Worksheet on the facing page. You can also download and make copies of the Alternative Thoughts Worksheet from *www.guilford.com/resick2-forms*. It might look complicated, but you have already learned and completed almost everything on the page. We'll break it into sections so that you can understand how it maps onto the processes you've already learned.

• **ABC.** The first two columns are the same as the ABC Worksheet you learned earlier. Write the event or situation in Section A. For now, this should be the most distressing traumatic event (name it—don't avoid by calling it "the event" or "the thing that happened"). As you eventually move on from evaluating your thoughts about the cause of your trauma, you may evaluate your stuck points that come up in everyday situations. In these cases, the more specific you can be on the worksheet about the event, the easier it will be to answer the questions, think about your patterns of thinking, and come up with a more balanced and fact-based thought.

Next, under B, write in one of your stuck points about that event (just one per

Alternative Thoughts Worksheet

A. Situation

Describe the event leading to the stuck point or unpleasant emotion(s).

B. Stuck point

Write your stuck point related to the situation in Section A. Rate your belief in this stuck point from 0 to 100%.

(How strongly do you believe this thought?)

C. Emotion(s)

Specify your emotion(s) (sad, angry, etc.) and rate how strongly you feel each emotion from 0 to 100%.

D. Exploring thoughts

Use the **exploring questions** to examine your automatic thought from Section B.

Consider whether the thought is balanced and factual or extreme.

Evidence against?

What information is not included?

All or none? Extreme?

Focused on just one piece of the event?

Questionable source of information?

Confusing possible with definite?

Based on feelings or facts?

E. Thinking patterns

Use the **thinking patterns** to decide whether this is one of the patterns and explain why.

Jumping to conclusions:

Ignoring important parts:

Oversimplifying/overgeneralizing:

Mind reading:

Emotional reasoning:

F. Alternative thought(s)

What else can you say instead of the thought in Section B? How else can you interpret the event instead of this thought? Rate your belief in the alternative thought(s) from 0 to 100%.

G. Re-rate old stuck point

Re-rate how much you now believe the stuck point in Section B from 0 to 100%.

H. Emotion(s)

Now what do you feel? Rate from 0 to 100%.

worksheet). If you started with B, the thought, make sure you go back and fill in A, the specific event. Now we're adding something new. Rate how much you believe that thought from 0 to 100%. When you were first starting out in this process, you might have believed it totally (100%) and assumed your thought was actually a fact. However, now that you can tell the difference between a fact and an opinion (your stuck point), you might not believe it completely anymore. The same applies for the emotions you feel when you think that stuck point.

In Section C, write down the emotion or emotions you feel when you think the stuck point (go back and look at the Identifying Emotions diagram on page 63 if you need to). Rating the strength of your emotions is also new to this worksheet. Rate how strongly you feel each emotion on a scale from 0 to 100%. In the beginning, you may have rated everything as 100%. Now it's possible that your emotions may have lessened.

• **Exploring thoughts.** Next, in the D section are abbreviations of all of the exploring questions from page 106 that you asked yourself earlier. If you need to, go back and look at the full questions as you answer them with regard to the stuck point in B. Try to answer as many as you can, and instead of just saying "Yes" or "No," write down enough so that you can look back later and understand why the answer was yes or no.

• **Thinking patterns.** In Section E are the thinking patterns that you were working on in the last chapter on page 125–131. Does this stuck point represent any of those patterns? If so, write down how this stuck point fits into one or more of the patterns.

• **Adding an alternative thought.** The final column includes important new skills we are adding in this chapter. This is an opportunity to add a different thought that may be more fact based or helpful. (Although you actually may have already practiced this skill too when you were completing the ABC Worksheet on page 93 if you answered the questions at the bottom of the worksheet "What can you tell yourself on such occasions in the future?") What else could you say instead of your stuck point after going through the steps on the worksheet? Is there something you can say that is more balanced and fact based than what you have been saying out of habit? Is there a way to think about the event that is more fair to yourself and the situation?

People often have a hard time figuring out what else they can say to themselves. Refer to the tip box on the facing page for ideas about how to write an alternative thought.

Ideally the alternative thought will be balanced (not an extreme statement), fact based, fair, and, importantly, one that you believe at least somewhat. Notice how you feel when you say the old thought and how you feel when you say the alternative thought. Try out different alternative thoughts to see if there is one in particular that you think is most accurate and helpful that you can repeat to yourself.

Now rate how much you believe this new thought from 0 to 100%. Write that number in the same box as your alternative thought (Section F). If you don't believe it at all, you should keep thinking about what would be an alternative thought you do believe, at least somewhat.

• **Rerating the original stuck point.** Next, in Section G, rate how much you now believe the original stuck point. Do you still believe it as much as you did at the beginning

Tips for Developing an Alternative Thought

⊃ A good starting point might be what you put under "evidence against." For example, if your stuck point was "If only I had fought harder, I could have stopped the assault" and your evidence against was "I fought as hard as I could"; "There were two of them and one of me"; and "If I had been able to fight harder, I might have been injured worse or killed," you could use one of these as your alternative thought, or you could summarize these points, and your alternative thought might be "I did the best I could and survived the assault."

⊃ It can help to say why you did what you did or what was actually realistic after you consider the full context of the event. You might say, "I didn't really have a choice because things happened so fast" or "I didn't intend for the car accident to happen. I was just trying to take a shortcut to work."

⊃ Another tip is to look for extreme words in your stuck point. If you have words or phrases like *should* or *must* or *every time,* can you soften those words so they are less extreme? The words *should* and *must* sound like commands. Are you being perfectionistic?

⊃ Is it even possible for something to happen or to do something "every time"? Does something happen *every* time or just sometimes? Likewise, is anything true of "everyone," or is it more accurate to say "some people"? If you can find even a single exception, then you could soften your language to "sometimes" or "some people." Would that small change feel different or change how you behave?

⊃ A final tip is to stop yourself from moving from one extreme to the other with your alternative thought: If your stuck point was "People will always hurt me," the alternative balanced thought is *not* "People will never hurt me." That would be too extreme on the opposite side. How about "It's possible that someone could hurt me, but it's unlikely that everyone is trying to hurt me"? How would that feel?

of the worksheet (in Section B)? Has it reduced at all now that you've considered the evidence? It's OK if you still believe the stuck point somewhat. You may have believed it 100% originally, so any reduction suggests that you now have multiple different ways to think about the event.

• **Rerating emotions.** Finally, in Section H, write in what emotions you feel now and how strongly you feel them when you think the alternative thought you came up with in Section F. Are they at the same intensity as they were at the beginning of the worksheet when you were thinking the stuck point (compared to what you put in Section C)? Sometimes the emotions don't just get less intense; sometimes they change entirely. If your emotion in Section C was guilty and you realize that it was someone else's fault, the guilt may reduce, but you also may start to feel angry that someone chose to hurt you that way. That is a natural emotion when someone else intends you harm. There may be natural emotions associated with accepting the traumatic event, such as grief and sadness. It's important to experience those natural emotions. They won't last forever, and you don't need to do something to stop them. Just let yourself feel whatever it is that you feel. They will eventually decrease if you let yourself feel them and don't block them by repeating your stuck points.

If there is no difference in your emotions when you change your thinking to the alternative thought, or if you don't believe the new statement, perhaps you should go over the worksheet some more and see if you can get any more helpful ideas. Remember to focus on the evidence against your stuck point. If the evidence against is factual, it can be the basis for an alternative thought. Remember also that this is not necessarily a skill that you were taught in school, so it takes practice. You'll need to continue to work on the stuck points about the cause of your traumas as long as you still have them. After you have worked through those stuck points, you can start to work on the ways you think about the present and future.

Don't worry if you don't believe the new thought fully yet or you think to yourself "I know that this alternative thought is true, but I still feel _____." You are in the middle of this program and in the middle of changing your thoughts, so your emotions might not have caught up with you yet. Once you come up with a good worksheet, you can read it over and over, reflecting on the reality of the event, until the alternative thought sounds more comfortable and realistic, true, or fair to you.

> ▶▶ To watch a video to review what you just read about the Alternative Thoughts Worksheet, go to the CPT Whiteboard Video Library (*http://cptforptsd.com/cpt-resources*) and watch the video called *How to Fill Out an Alternative Thoughts Worksheet*. You can also watch a video called *Alternative Thoughts Worksheet Example*.

 ## PRACTICE ASSIGNMENT

Use the Alternative Thoughts Worksheets to analyze at least one of your stuck points each day. Start with stuck points from your log about the cause of the traumatic events. Complete at least one Alternative Thoughts Worksheet each day until you are comfortable examining your stuck points with the questions and can develop alternative thoughts that you can use to counteract your unhelpful thoughts or until you have completed a week of practice.

Remember to focus on the stuck points that have kept you stuck in your PTSD, like self-blame, blaming people who didn't actually intend the harm, *if only*s or *shoulda–coulda–woulda* statements, if you still believe these. Also, continue to prioritize your stuck points about your index trauma. As you work through your stuck points about that event, you can also start to do worksheets on stuck points related to other traumas that you may have experienced. If you notice any new stuck points, remember to add them to your Stuck Point Log (page 56).

There are some example Alternative Thoughts Worksheets that have already been completed on pages 141–142 for you to refer to. These are followed by a number of blank worksheets (pages 143–149).

A. Situation	B. Stuck point	C. Emotion(s)	D. Exploring thoughts	E. Thinking patterns	F. Alternative thought(s)	G. Re-rate old stuck point	H. Emotion(s)
Describe the event leading to the stuck point or unpleasant emotion(s).	Write your stuck point related to the situation in Section A. Rate your belief in this stuck point from 0 to 100%. (How strongly do you believe this thought?)	Specify your emotion(s) (sad, angry, etc.) and rate how strongly you feel each emotion from 0 to 100%.	Use the **exploring questions** to examine your automatic thought from Section B. Consider whether the thought is balanced and factual or extreme.	Use the **thinking patterns** to decide whether this is one of the patterns and explain why.	What else can you say instead of the thought in Section B? How else can you interpret the event instead of this thought? Rate your belief in the alternative thought(s) from 0 to 100%.	Re-rate how much you now believe the stuck point in Section B from 0 to 100%.	Now what do you feel? Rate from 0 to 100%.
My husband dying in the building collapse.	I should have listened to my gut that something was wrong that day and not let him go to work. 90%	Guilt 100% Regret 100%	Evidence against? I didn't know the building was going to collapse. What information is not included? I didn't know why I had a bad feeling. Also I have had bad feelings before and sometimes it was nothing or something minor. All or none? Extreme? Saying "should have."	Jumping to conclusions:	I wish I knew that this event was going to happen and could have kept my husband safe, but realistically speaking, I didn't have enough information then to act on. I had a bad feeling, but it didn't tell me what to do, and it's unrealistic to think I could have kept my husband home. 70%	25%	Sad 80% Regret 25%
		Focused on just one piece of the event? Focused on the gut feeling. Questionable source of information? I guess it's based on hindsight. I'm looking back now saying what "I should have" done then based on the outcome.	Ignoring important parts: Even if I had tried to convince him to stay home from work, he probably would have gone anyway. He had important meetings that day. Oversimplifying/overgeneralizing:			
			Confusing possible with definite? Based on feelings or facts? Definitely feelings.	Mind reading:			
				Emotional reasoning: Definitely based on emotions. I feel guilty and go back to my gut at the time, but I didn't have any facts.			

Example Alternative Thoughts Worksheet

A. Situation	B. Stuck point	C. Emotion(s)	D. Exploring thoughts	E. Thinking patterns	F. Alternative thought(s)	G. Re-rate old stuck point	H. Emotion(s)
Describe the event leading to the stuck point or unpleasant emotion(s).	Write your stuck point related to the situation in Section A. Rate your belief in this stuck point from 0 to 100%. (How strongly do you believe this thought?)	Specify your emotion(s) (sad, angry, etc.) and rate how strongly you feel each emotion from 0 to 100%.	Use the **exploring questions** to examine your automatic thought from Section B. Consider whether the thought is balanced and factual or extreme.	Use the **thinking patterns** to decide whether this is one of the patterns and explain why.	What else can you say instead of the thought in Section B? How else can you interpret the event instead of this thought? Rate your belief in the alternative thought(s) from 0 to 100%.	Re-rate how much you now believe the stuck point in Section B from 0 to 100%.	Now what do you feel? Rate from 0 to 100%.
Seeing a child who was murdered as part of my job as a police officer.	*Things like this aren't supposed to happen to innocent children.* 100%		*Evidence against? I guess ideally murder wouldn't happen to anyone—children or otherwise. But it does happen.* *What information is not included?* *All or none? Extreme? It is exaggerated to say that it is not "supposed to" happen as if there is a universal rule that children will never be harmed.*	Jumping to conclusions:	*Ideally children (and adults) would be safe, but that is not always the case. Sometimes bad things happen or people do harmful things, and it is not always fair who suffers the consequences.* 100%	20%	*Angry 50%* *Sad 50%*
		Angry 75% Confused 80%	*Focused on just one piece of the event?* *Focused on their being children.* *Questionable source of information?* *This belief comes from moral views that children are to be protected. That is an ideal, but that does not mean that it always works that way.* *Confusing possible with definite?* *Based on feelings or facts?* *Based on my feelings of outrage.*	Ignoring important parts: *When I say that this is not supposed to happen to children, I am leaving out that unfortunately things like this happen frequently. Children are vulnerable, and so they are often the victims of crimes. That has been the case since the beginning of time.* Oversimplifying/overgeneralizing: *Assuming that children should always be safe, which is not realistic or possible.* Mind reading: Emotional reasoning: *It feels so wrong and devastating when things like this happen.*			

Alternative Thoughts Worksheet

A. Situation	B. Stuck point	C. Emotion(s)	D. Exploring thoughts	E. Thinking patterns	F. Alternative thought(s)
Describe the event leading to the stuck point or unpleasant emotion(s).	Write your stuck point related to the situation in Section A. Rate your belief in this stuck point from 0 to 100%. (How strongly do you believe this thought?)	Specify your emotion(s) (sad, angry, etc.) and rate how strongly you feel each emotion from 0 to 100%.	Use the **exploring questions** to examine your automatic thought from Section B. Consider whether the thought is balanced and factual or extreme.	Use the **thinking patterns** to decide whether this is one of the patterns and explain why.	What else can you say instead of the thought in Section B? How else can you interpret the event instead of this thought? Rate your belief in the alternative thought(s) from 0 to 100%.
			Evidence against?	Jumping to conclusions:	
			What information is not included?	Ignoring important parts:	
			All or none? Extreme?	Oversimplifying/overgeneralizing:	
			Focused on just one piece of the event?		
			Questionable source of information?	Mind reading:	
			Confusing possible with definite?		**G. Re-rate old stuck point** Re-rate how much you now believe the stuck point in Section B from 0 to 100%.
			Based on feelings or facts?	Emotional reasoning:	**H. Emotion(s)** Now what do you feel? Rate from 0 to 100%.

From *Getting Unstuck from PTSD* by Patricia A. Resick, Shannon Wiltsey Stirman, and Stefanie T. LoSavio. Copyright © 2023 The Guilford Press. Purchasers of this book can photocopy and/or download additional copies of this worksheet at *www.guilford.com/resick2-forms* for personal use or use with clients; see copyright page for details.

Alternative Thoughts Worksheet

A. Situation	B. Stuck point	D. Exploring thoughts	E. Thinking patterns	F. Alternative thought(s)
Describe the event leading to the stuck point or unpleasant emotion(s).	Write your stuck point related to the situation in Section A. Rate your belief in this stuck point from 0 to 100%. (How strongly do you believe this thought?)	Use the **exploring questions** to examine your automatic thought from Section B. Consider whether the thought is balanced and factual or extreme.	Use the **thinking patterns** to decide whether this is one of the patterns and explain why.	What else can you say instead of the thought in Section B? How else can you interpret the event instead of this thought? Rate your belief in the alternative thought(s) from 0 to 100%.
		Evidence against?	Jumping to conclusions:	
		What information is not included?	Ignoring important parts:	
		All or none? Extreme?		
		Focused on just one piece of the event?	Oversimplifying/overgeneralizing:	G. Re-rate old stuck point
	C. Emotion(s) Specify your emotion(s) (sad, angry, etc.) and rate how strongly you feel each emotion from 0 to 100%.	Questionable source of information?	Mind reading:	Re-rate how much you now believe the stuck point in Section B from 0 to 100%.
		Confusing possible with definite?		
		Based on feelings or facts?	Emotional reasoning:	**H. Emotion(s)** Now what do you feel? Rate from 0 to 100%.

Alternative Thoughts Worksheet

A. Situation	B. Stuck point	C. Emotion(s)	D. Exploring thoughts	E. Thinking patterns	F. Alternative thought(s)
Describe the event leading to the stuck point or unpleasant emotion(s).	Write your stuck point related to the situation in Section A. Rate your belief in this stuck point from 0 to 100%. (How strongly do you believe this thought?)	Specify your emotion(s) (sad, angry, etc.) and rate how strongly you feel each emotion from 0 to 100%.	Use the exploring questions to examine your automatic thought from Section B. Consider whether the thought is balanced and factual or extreme.	Use the thinking patterns to decide whether this is one of the patterns and explain why.	What else can you say instead of the thought in Section B? How else can you interpret the event instead of this thought? Rate your belief in the alternative thought(s) from 0 to 100%.
			Evidence against?	Jumping to conclusions:	
			What information is not included?	Ignoring important parts:	
			All or none? Extreme?		
			Focused on just one piece of the event?	Oversimplifying/overgeneralizing:	
			Questionable source of information?	Mind reading:	**G. Re-rate old stuck point** Re-rate how much you now believe the stuck point in Section B from 0 to 100%.
			Confusing possible with definite?		
			Based on feelings or facts?	Emotional reasoning:	**H. Emotion(s)** Now what do you feel? Rate from 0 to 100%.

Alternative Thoughts Worksheet

A. Situation	B. Stuck point	C. Emotion(s)	D. Exploring thoughts	E. Thinking patterns	F. Alternative thought(s)	G. Re-rate old stuck point	H. Emotion(s)
Describe the event leading to the stuck point or unpleasant emotion(s).	Write your stuck point related to the situation in Section A. Rate your belief in this stuck point from 0 to 100%. (How strongly do you believe this thought?)	Specify your emotion(s) (sad, angry, etc.) and rate how strongly you feel each emotion from 0 to 100%.	Use the **exploring questions** to examine your automatic thought from Section B. Consider whether the thought is balanced and factual or extreme.	Use the **thinking patterns** to decide whether this is one of the patterns and explain why.	What else can you say instead of the thought in Section B? How else can you interpret the event instead of this thought? Rate your belief in the alternative thought(s) from 0 to 100%.	Re-rate how much you now believe the stuck point in Section B from 0 to 100%.	Now what do you feel? Rate from 0 to 100%.
			Evidence against?	Jumping to conclusions:			
			What information is not included?	Ignoring important parts:			
			All or none? Extreme?	Oversimplifying/overgeneralizing:			
			Focused on just one piece of the event?				
			Questionable source of information?	Mind reading:			
			Confusing possible with definite?				
			Based on feelings or facts?	Emotional reasoning:			

Alternative Thoughts Worksheet

A. Situation	B. Stuck point	C. Emotion(s)	D. Exploring thoughts	E. Thinking patterns	F. Alternative thought(s)
Describe the event leading to the stuck point or unpleasant emotion(s).	Write your stuck point related to the situation in Section A. Rate your belief in this stuck point from 0 to 100%. (How strongly do you believe this thought?)	Specify your emotion(s) (sad, angry, etc.) and rate how strongly you feel each emotion from 0 to 100%.	Use the **exploring questions** to examine your automatic thought from Section B. Consider whether the thought is balanced and factual or extreme.	Use the **thinking patterns** to decide whether this is one of the patterns and explain why.	What else can you say instead of the thought in Section B? How else can you interpret the event instead of this thought? Rate your belief in the alternative thought(s) from 0 to 100%.
			Evidence against?	Jumping to conclusions:	
			What information is not included?	Ignoring important parts:	
			All or none? Extreme?		
			Focused on just one piece of the event?	Oversimplifying/overgeneralizing:	
			Questionable source of information?	Mind reading:	G. Re-rate old stuck point — Re-rate how much you now believe the stuck point in Section B from 0 to 100%.
			Confusing possible with definite?		
			Based on feelings or facts?	Emotional reasoning:	H. Emotion(s) — Now what do you feel? Rate from 0 to 100%.

Alternative Thoughts Worksheet

A. Situation	B. Stuck point	D. Exploring thoughts	E. Thinking patterns	F. Alternative thought(s)
Describe the event leading to the stuck point or unpleasant emotion(s).	Write your stuck point related to the situation in Section A. Rate your belief in this stuck point from 0 to 100%. (How strongly do you believe this thought?)	Use the **exploring questions** to examine your automatic thought from Section B. Consider whether the thought is balanced and factual or extreme.	Use the **thinking patterns** to decide whether this is one of the patterns and explain why.	What else can you say instead of the thought in Section B? How else can you interpret the event instead of this thought? Rate your belief in the alternative thought(s) from 0 to 100%.
		Evidence against?	Jumping to conclusions:	
		What information is not included?	Ignoring important parts:	
		All or none? Extreme?		
		Focused on just one piece of the event?	Oversimplifying/overgeneralizing:	
	C. Emotion(s) Specify your emotion(s) (sad, angry, etc.) and rate how strongly you feel each emotion from 0 to 100%.	Questionable source of information?	Mind reading:	**G. Re-rate old stuck point** Re-rate how much you now believe the stuck point in Section B from 0 to 100%.
		Confusing possible with definite?		
		Based on feelings or facts?	Emotional reasoning:	**H. Emotion(s)** Now what do you feel? Rate from 0 to 100%.

Alternative Thoughts Worksheet

A. Situation	B. Stuck point	D. Exploring thoughts	E. Thinking patterns	F. Alternative thought(s)
Describe the event leading to the stuck point or unpleasant emotion(s).	Write your stuck point related to the situation in Section A. Rate your belief in this stuck point from 0 to 100%. (How strongly do you believe this thought?)	Use the **exploring questions** to examine your automatic thought from Section B. Consider whether the thought is balanced and factual or extreme.	Use the **thinking patterns** to decide whether this is one of the patterns and explain why.	What else can you say instead of the thought in Section B? How else can you interpret the event instead of this thought? Rate your belief in the alternative thought(s) from 0 to 100%.
		Evidence against?	Jumping to conclusions:	
		What information is not included?	Ignoring important parts:	
		All or none? Extreme?	Oversimplifying/overgeneralizing:	
		Focused on just one piece of the event?		
		Questionable source of information?	Mind reading:	**G. Re-rate old stuck point** Re-rate how much you now believe the stuck point in Section B from 0 to 100%.
		Confusing possible with definite?		
	C. Emotion(s) Specify your emotion(s) (sad, angry, etc.) and rate how strongly you feel each emotion from 0 to 100%.	Based on feelings or facts?	Emotional reasoning:	**H. Emotion(s)** Now what do you feel? Rate from 0 to 100%.

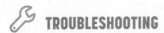 **TROUBLESHOOTING**

This worksheet seems too complicated.

Try covering up the worksheet with a blank piece of paper. Now slide the paper to the right to uncover just the first two columns on the left side. Does this look familiar? That's the ABC Worksheet that you have done many times. The only difference is that now we are asking you to rate how much you believe the stuck point and how strongly you feel your emotions. The next column over is the Exploring Questions Worksheet. You've already practiced this skill, too. The seven questions are summarized with just a few words to fit into the column, but you can go back to Chapter 8 (pages 107–109) to look at the actual questions and examples. The next column reflects the work you did in Chapter 9 on the Thinking Patterns Worksheet (pages 125–131). The only thing that is new on this worksheet is the column on the far right in which you write down an alternative thought, rate how strongly you believe it, how strongly you now believe the old stuck point, and what emotions and how strongly you feel them after completing the worksheet. Look at the example worksheets on pages 141–142 and use the previous chapters to help you complete this worksheet. It will get easier the more you practice, and it doesn't have to be perfect to get the benefits of practicing these skills!

I can't come up with a good alternative thought.

The seeds for a good alternative thought are in your answers to the questions. Look at what you put under the "evidence against" your stuck point or "not including all the information." You might also realize that you have been focusing on something that was not factual. If you found a number of facts that make your stuck point not one hundred percent true, you can focus on that to think about what else you could say to yourself instead of the stuck point. You can also look back over the worksheet and think about what you would say to a friend who had that experience. Try writing that down and seeing how it makes you feel to say that to yourself.

I can't change what happened to me. It happened.

It's important to note that the purpose of the worksheet is not to question what happened to you. You are correct—it happened, and the goal is to accept it rather than to try to mentally undo it after the fact. What you are examining are your *thoughts* about what happened, such as why it happened and what or who caused the event, and what it means to and about you now. We don't question or change situations or facts, only *interpretations* of situations that may not be one hundred percent accurate and that might keep you stuck in PTSD. In other words, we are not trying to get rid of the event or the memory but only the power it has over you.

I'm not sure where to put my answers.

Some of the questions are asking similar things. You may not be sure which place to write your ideas. Often you could put the same point under "evidence against" or "not including all the information." Sometimes the same idea fits for "oversimplifying/overgeneralizing" and "emotional reasoning." You could put your answers anywhere that makes sense to you. Remember that the worksheets are just a tool for you to evaluate your thinking.

Do I have to answer every question?

Answer as many as you can and try to write in explanations instead of just "Yes" or "No." However, you may not need to answer all of the questions or thinking patterns, just the ones that fit the stuck point. Sometimes a question doesn't apply to a particular stuck point. Also, if you get stuck, you can move on to the next question.

What if I still believe my stuck point?

It's not unusual to still believe your stuck point the first time you do a worksheet on it, but hopefully you are starting to consider more facts and other ways of looking at it. Keep working on it with more worksheets. Also, you may ask yourself if there is some reason you are hanging on to that thought. Is it part of your automatic core belief? Is there an even scarier idea underneath that you are protecting? For example, do you want to hold on to the blame because if you let go of it you'll think that you don't have any control over your life or over whether something bad will happen again? If so, write that second stuck point on your log ("If I couldn't have prevented it, it means I don't have any control over what happens") and start working on it.

What if my emotions don't change?

Emotions can change in type or strength. You might not notice that you are not as scared or ashamed as you were before. Or you might notice that you feel a similar emotion but for a different reason and with a different intensity or direction. For example, you might go from feeling guilty and angry at yourself to angry at the perpetrator. Or you might have originally felt sadness (and shame) thinking the stuck point "I was abused because I was unlovable" but now just feel sadness thinking the alternative thought "I was abused because they chose to abuse me." Although both thoughts may lead to sadness, the sadness from the alternative thought will dissipate in intensity over time if you let yourself feel it. Sadness that a trauma happened is a natural emotion, so it makes sense you would still feel sad. Letting yourself feel the sadness will help you move toward recovery. Remember, even if you always feel some sadness because what happened involved a loss of something or someone important to you, it will become less intense, and more of a quiet sadness over time, and you may notice that you become more able to enjoy positive emotions in addition to feeling sadness than you are able to when the traumatic memories weren't processed. If your emotions don't change at all, go back and consider the questions again and see if you can come up with a more helpful alternative thought. Perhaps the one you wrote as an alternative is not very different from the original stuck point. Find something that is balanced (not extreme), is based on facts, and that you believe at least somewhat. See if you can write something that seems to be fair or accurate based on all of the information about the event. It may take a while for your emotions to catch up with your thinking.

(PTSD Checklist)

Complete the PTSD Checklist to track your symptoms as you complete this book. Be sure to complete this measure on the same index event each time. When the instructions and questions refer to a "stressful experience," remember that that is your index event—the worst event that you are working on first.

Write in here the trauma that you are working on first: _____

Complete this PTSD Checklist with reference to that event.

Instructions: Below is a list of problems that people sometimes have in response to a very stressful experience. Please read each problem carefully, and then circle one of the numbers to the right to indicate how much you have been bothered by that problem *in the past week*.

In the past week, how much were you bothered by:	Not at all	A little bit	Mod- erately	Quite a bit	Extremely
1. Repeated, disturbing, and unwanted memories of the stressful experience?	0	1	2	3	4
2. Repeated, disturbing dreams of the stressful experience?	0	1	2	3	4
3. Suddenly feeling or acting as if the stressful experience were actually happening again (*as if you were actually back there reliving it*)?	0	1	2	3	4
4. Feeling very upset when something reminded you of the stressful experience?	0	1	2	3	4
5. Having strong physical reactions when something reminded you of the stressful experience (*for example, heart pounding, trouble breathing, sweating*)?	0	1	2	3	4
6. Avoiding memories, thoughts, or feelings related to the stressful experience?	0	1	2	3	4
7. Avoiding external reminders of the stressful experience (*for example, people, places, conversations, activities, objects, or situations*)?	0	1	2	3	4
8. Trouble remembering important parts of the stressful experience (not due to head injury or substances)?	0	1	2	3	4
9. Having strong negative beliefs about yourself, other people, or the world (*for example, having thoughts such as I am bad, There is something seriously wrong with me, No one can be trusted, or The world is completely dangerous*)?	0	1	2	3	4
10. Blaming yourself or someone else (who didn't intend the outcome) for the stressful experience or what happened after it?	0	1	2	3	4
11. Having strong negative feelings, such as fear, horror, anger, guilt, or shame?	0	1	2	3	4
12. Loss of interest in activities that you used to enjoy?	0	1	2	3	4
13. Feeling distant or cut off from other people?	0	1	2	3	4
14. Trouble experiencing positive feelings (*for example, being unable to feel happiness or have loving feelings for people close to you*)?	0	1	2	3	4
15. Irritable behavior, angry outbursts, or acting aggressively?	0	1	2	3	4
16. Taking too many risks or doing things that could cause you harm?	0	1	2	3	4
17. Being "super alert" or watchful or on guard?	0	1	2	3	4
18. Feeling jumpy or easily startled?	0	1	2	3	4
19. Having difficulty concentrating?	0	1	2	3	4
20. Trouble falling or staying asleep?	0	1	2	3	4

Add up the total and write it here: _____

~~~~~~~~~~~~~~~~~~~~ Reflecting on Your Progress ~~~~~~~~~~~~~~~~~~~~

Now is a good time to pause and reflect on your progress so far. Take the time to complete the PTSD Checklist and look over the total scores from week to week on the Graph for Tracking Your Weekly Scores from page 24 to see if you notice any changes in your symptom level. Are you seeing improvement in your symptoms as evidenced by decreasing scores? Are you noticing other changes in your everyday life? For example, have you been going places you've been avoiding or reacting to people and situations differently than you used to? Do you feel different when you think about the traumatic event? There are many different ways that you might notice progress.

Also, look over your Stuck Point Log. In particular, go over the stuck points you have about the traumatic event, such as why it happened, who is to blame for it, whether it could have been prevented, and the like. Do you still believe these thoughts as much as you did when you first wrote them down? If there are any stuck points on your log that you no longer believe, you can cross them out. Congratulate yourself for any progress you have made thinking through your beliefs about the event! If you still believe these stuck points, or still think they are at least somewhat true, you can leave them on your log and continue to work on them in the chapters ahead. Don't worry if you still believe most of your stuck points. There will be lots of opportunities to continue making progress on your stuck points and symptoms over the next chapters.

If You Are Not Noticing Change

First, it's important to remember that you have probably been thinking one way for a long time, so it will take practice to develop a new way of thinking. If you have noticed that you have tendencies to think the same way across situations (same stuck points or patterns of thinking), you may have a **core belief** that is so ingrained that you don't have to consciously think it anymore. It's just an assumption that seems like **truth**. A core belief cannot be changed with just one worksheet. It's too big. Even if you believe on some level that your stuck point isn't true, it might still "feel" true. The good news is that your head and your heart used to agree that your stuck point was true. If you've started changing your thinking, your feelings might take some time to catch up, because we can all have a tendency toward emotional reasoning or acting out of habit rather than looking at the facts. You may have to complete many more worksheets or catch yourself and remind yourself of the work you've done that's changed your belief until the stuck point doesn't sound or feel like "truth" anymore.

Also take a moment to ask yourself whether you are working on the trauma, or the part of the trauma, that is hardest for you. Sometimes it's difficult to face something that you feel a lot of fear, guilt, or shame about. However, until you do, you'll notice limited progress. By now you have practiced and built up some skills. Try applying them to any self-blame-related stuck points about the memory that haunts you the most, or the trauma you have the most nightmares about, or the aspect of the trauma that you have the most shame about. Sometimes, like in the example on page 154, taking a closer look at the stuck points that bring up the most guilt or shame can bring to light some important information, or things you haven't considered, which might change how you've been thinking about the event and what it means about you. It is courageous to do this work, and it isn't easy. If there are supportive people in your life who you can talk with as you face these things, you might want to let them know you are going to be doing an especially challenging part of your PTSD recovery work and let them know how they can support you. Note that you can ask for support without telling people all of the details about what happened if you want or need to keep those details private. They can support you without knowing everything.

> Michael was sexually molested repeatedly by an uncle when he was young, and physically abused by his parents. He had started working on the physical abuse, but noticed that his PTSD was not improving, even though he was working through the book and completing a worksheet every day. He didn't believe the abuse was his fault anymore, but he still felt ashamed. Michael began to realize that he felt most deeply ashamed about the sexual molestation, so he started completing worksheets on that trauma. The event he felt most ashamed of was a time that he experienced an orgasm during the abuse. He was also ashamed that he would get erections at times when he was molested. He added to his Stuck Point Log "I must have liked what happened" and "I am a pervert." However, physical arousal can occur whenever we encounter sexually relevant stimuli or our bodies are touched. Our brains associate some things with sexual activity, such as seeing certain parts of the body or experiencing certain types of stimulation, even if they are not things that we find enjoyable during unwanted sexual experiences. Our physical responses can be separate from our emotional responses. Physical arousal is not the same thing as enjoyment. We also know that sometimes during fight–flight–freeze reactions, blood can flow to all of our extremities, and for men, erections can occur. It's a physiological reality for all genders that some types of stimulation can result in orgasm, even if the person experiencing it does not feel that they are enjoying it physically or emotionally. Once Michael realized that, he began to let go of the shame he felt. He realized that his physical response didn't actually mean that he had enjoyed or wanted the molestation to happen. He was a child, and he had been very confused and overwhelmed by the experience. But looking at it as an adult, he recognized that he did nothing wrong. He felt a sense of relief, but also some sadness about what had happened to him, and appropriate anger at his uncle for what he had done. After he let himself feel these natural emotions, he noticed that he began to feel better.

If you are still experiencing intrusive memories, flashbacks, or nightmares, are they about the event that you have been working on, or is there another traumatic event that bothers you more? If you did not start with the traumatic event that is having the most impact on you, you may need to think about what stuck points you have about the other event. Are they the same or different? If they are different stuck points specific to the event that you are having flashbacks or nightmares about, make sure to get them on your Stuck Point Log and start working on them.

It also goes without saying that if you have skipped ahead and not practiced using the skills already covered, it would be no surprise if you are still struggling with your PTSD symptoms. Are there any ways that you may be avoiding? Have you been procrastinating on doing the worksheets every day because it's so difficult to face your memories or because you're worried you won't do them perfectly? Have you been reading the text but not writing on the worksheets? Remind yourself of your reasons for working on your PTSD, and about your goals for yourself. Make sure you have practiced the worksheets in previous chapters and that you have not skipped over your stuck points about why the trauma happened. If you have, go back and work on those now.

On that note, do you have any other stuck points that you still haven't worked on yet about why the trauma happened, whether it could have been prevented, or whether it was fair? Try to think about what is really keeping you stuck. Do you still feel guilty, regretful, ashamed, or angry at yourself? If so, ask yourself why and then continue to use the skills to work on the thought that comes up. Here are some examples of common stuck points people need to do worksheets on to make progress. Check off any that you might still need to work on:

- ❑ The event could have been prevented.
- ❑ It's my fault the event happened.
- ❑ The event happened because of something about me.
- ❑ I let the event happen.
- ❑ I must have done something to deserve the event.
- ❑ If I had been more careful/observant, it wouldn't have happened.
- ❑ I should have said or done something different.
- ❑ I brought it on myself.

Go back to the questions in Chapter 7 starting on page 79 to help you address any of these types of beliefs. Sometimes people also get stuck in PTSD because of beliefs about fairness or how the world is "supposed" to work. Do you have any stuck points like these that you haven't worked on yet?

- ❑ Things like this aren't supposed to happen.
- ❑ Life should be fair.
- ❑ Bad events are always preventable.
- ❑ It shouldn't have happened again. All of that was supposed to be behind me.
- ❑ All events have a clear cause.
- ❑ There has to be a good reason that it happened.

For these types of stuck points, it's important to consider if that is in fact how the world always works or if that's simply how it would ideally work. Go back and reflect on the questions starting on page 100. Then you may need to feel your natural emotions, like sadness.

Finally, if you have been examining a stuck point and feel like you're not getting anywhere, consider rewording the stuck point. Maybe if you word it differently (for example, instead of "I let it happen" you could try working on "I should have yelled for help"), you will think of new ways to look at it that you haven't before. Also check to make sure that your stuck points are about a specific event ("If I had been in a different position, I could have saved my friend") and are not too big or vague ("It's the military's fault"). Trying to take on a big concept instead of a specific event is more difficult to make progress on.

Difficulty Letting Go of Stuck Points

Are there any stuck points about the traumatic event that you did worksheets on, considered the evidence for, and tried to think up alternative thoughts for, but you're still feeling stuck on? Or maybe there are stuck points that you now know "logically" are not realistic but you still "feel" like they are true? This is quite common.

First of all, your stuck points are usually ways that you've been thinking for a long time, so they may have become automatic ways of thinking. It can sometimes take a lot of practice looking at the situation from a new angle to have a different way of thinking compete with the old way. So keep going over the evidence and reminding yourself of the facts of the situation. You can even do another worksheet to reexamine the same stuck point again.

If you find that no matter how many times you go over the facts of the situation it's still hard to let go of the old way of thinking, consider the following:

What would it mean to give up the stuck point? What would it mean if the stuck point were not realistic or true?

_____

_____

_____

_____

What is an alternative possibility, and what would it mean if that were true?

_____

_____

_____

_____

How would you feel if you believed one of your alternative thoughts instead of the stuck point? Would any emotions come up that are hard to face?

_____

_____

Sometimes when a stuck point is difficult to let go of it's because thinking something different might actually seem worse. Consider the following example:

Lisa's teenage daughter was driving home from a party one evening when she got into a car accident and was killed. Lisa has been blaming herself for her daughter's death, thinking "I never should have let her go out that night. I could have prevented the accident by keeping her home." Lisa worked hard to consider the facts of the situation, what she knew at the time when she agreed to let her daughter go out, what her intention was, and considering how it was a case of hindsight bias. However, no matter how much Lisa considered these facts, she just kept thinking "But if I hadn't let her go out that night, she would still be alive." In other words, Lisa was struggling to let go of the idea that she could have prevented the accident somehow. She also started being even more protective of her other children, especially with them getting older, and they were missing opportunities to try new things and grow.

Lisa considered the questions above as follows:

What would it mean to give up the stuck point? What would mean if the stuck point were not realistic or true?

> If it's not realistic that I would have kept her home,
> then that means I couldn't have prevented it.

What would it mean to think something different?

> If I started thinking "I couldn't have prevented it,"
> it would mean that I can't always prevent bad things from happening.

How would you feel if you believed one of your alternative thoughts instead of the stuck point? Would any emotions come up that are hard to face?

> This way of thinking makes me feel scared. I don't like thinking that I can't
> control or prevent things from happening to my kids. I wish I could keep all
> my kids safe at all times. But I guess that's not always possible.

In this case, Lisa was taking on the blame for her daughter's accident because feeling the guilt was in a way better than feeling the fear that something bad could happen to her other children. It makes sense because for someone who has already faced trauma, the worst thing to imagine is that more trauma could happen. We would all rather believe that "As long as I don't make the same mistakes again, nothing like that will ever happen again." But is that realistic and true? It's a difficult fact to face that we don't have full control over what happens to us or our loved ones. In this case, Lisa faced the difficult reality that not only is it unrealistic that she could have prevented her daughter's accident but more generally, she can't prevent all bad things from happening. Of course, it is extremely unlikely that a trauma like her daughter's accident would happen again.

Consider another example:

Ahmed has been thinking about his friend who was killed during violence in his home country. He has often blamed himself and thought "I should have been there" and "If I were there that day, I could have protected him." Ahmed has done a lot of work to go over the facts. He has recognized that he couldn't be in all places at once and that even if he were there, he wouldn't necessarily have been able to save his friend, and he might have been hurt or killed, too. So, Ahmed has concluded that, logically, he couldn't have done anything, yet he was still feeling stuck.

Here are Ahmed's answers to one of the questions above:

What would it mean to give up the stuck point? What would it mean if the stuck point were not realistic or true?

> I know that the stuck point is not realistic. I think if I really gave up the idea that I could have done something to save him, I would feel less guilty. But maybe if I feel better and move on with my life, I am a bad friend. Like I am forgetting him and not honoring his memory.

In this case, Ahmed discovers that behind his original stuck point are more stuck points that are keeping him stuck in PTSD—namely, he is thinking "If I move on with my life, then I am a bad friend," and "If I feel better, I will forget my friend." These are more thoughts that Ahmed can evaluate with the questions and worksheets in this book. For example, he might consider whether continuing to suffer with PTSD is the best way to honor his friend or if there are other ways to do that. He can think about how he would hope his friends would live out their lives if he died early or unexpectedly. He might also consider what it means to be a good friend and whether self-blame is the best way to be a friend, or if he has already done many things in his friendships that would make people consider him to be a good friend.

Consider any stuck points you have had trouble letting go of to see if any of these problems are keeping you stuck. Then go back and reevaluate the stuck point.

Here are some common examples of stuck points that sometimes prevent people from letting go of self-blame and blame of others who did not directly cause the trauma:

❑ If I stop blaming myself/stop having PTSD, I will forget about [someone who died].

❑ I can't move on with my life because others who were involved didn't get to move on with theirs.

❑ I can't place the blame on the perpetrator because it's wrong to speak ill of the dead.

❑ I can't place the blame on (or be angry at) my parents because I must always honor my parents.

❑ I should always forgive. It's wrong to be angry.

❑ If I move forward with my life, it means I'm saying it's OK that the trauma happened.

If any of these ring true for you, do a worksheet on them. They are also stuck points.

On the other hand, here are some common examples of uncomfortable but likely true thoughts that sometimes hold people back from changing their stuck points because these facts are so difficult to accept:

❑ Considering the facts of your trauma might lead you to conclude "It just wasn't fair." Most likely, no, it wasn't.

- This is uncomfortable because it means life isn't always fair. This means that bad things can happen even when you don't do anything to deserve them. Think about how a tornado might demolish one house and then skip the next.

❑ Considering the facts of your trauma might lead you to conclude "I did everything I could and it still happened."

- This might be an unsettling thought because it means not all bad events are preventable.

❑ Considering the facts of your trauma might lead you to conclude "It wasn't my fault."

- This might be an unsettling thought, because it means you don't have full control over what happens to you.

❑ Considering the facts of your trauma might lead you to conclude "It wasn't something about me that caused it. It happened just because they wanted it to."

- This might be an uncomfortable thought because if it wasn't something about you (something that you can understand or control), then bad events can happen unexpectedly and you might not always be able to predict when or why they will happen or control what others do. You might have been the occasion but not the cause of the event (wrong place, wrong time).

❑ Considering the facts of the trauma might lead you to conclude "There wasn't a good reason that it happened."

- This might be an uncomfortable thought because, if there wasn't a good reason that this event happened, then sometimes events happen unexpectedly and for no good reason.

If any of these are thoughts you have, consider that these are likely true statements. These thoughts are uncomfortable because they highlight that sometimes events can be unpredictable, unforeseeable, and uncontrollable, and happen without good reason. No one likes to think about the world that way because we all would like to believe that we have control over what happens to us. But what do you think? Is that realistic all the time?

What emotion do you feel when you let yourself think these thoughts? Sadness? Grief? Perhaps some fear? Keep in mind that the fact that something bad *could* possibly happen again does not mean it's likely. Sit with the emotions that come up without immediately pushing them away. If you can face these thoughts and emotions, it will likely be easier to let go of unhelpful stuck points. In upcoming chapters we look more closely at living life even though we don't have the ability to control everything that happens.

When you have worked through these roadblocks, go back and reevaluate your original stuck points to see if you can make more progress.

If You Have Made Progress Reaching Your Goals

If you have made progress working through your Stuck Point Log (page 56) and your symptoms have decreased, that's terrific! People vary in how much CPT they need to reach their goals. Keep tracking your progress working through your stuck points and on the PTSD Checklist. If you have finished working on your stuck points about why the worst trauma happened and you want to move on to stuck points about why another trauma happened, you can do so. You can also start to move on to evaluating the more general beliefs about the present and future. If your score on the PTSD Checklist gets below 20, you may want to assess whether you have worked on all of the stuck points you need to and are ready to move toward wrapping up. Whenever you're ready, you can go to the section called "Planning for the Conclusion of CPT" on page 264. However, there is no rush. You can keep reviewing the chapters if you are finding them helpful.

Overall, there is no "right" number of weeks to complete this book; everyone is different. But tracking your progress on the PTSD Checklist and with your stuck points will help you figure out where you still need to spend time and to plan for the rest of your program.

Marcus had one major trauma to work on but no other issues. He started to realize that the traumatic event was unavoidable when he completed the Exploring Questions Worksheet. By the time he completed several Alternative Thoughts Worksheets, he had produced enough evidence to convince himself his stuck point was not accurate or helpful and found a good alternative thought. By then his score on the PTSD Checklist was 4 and he had crossed off all of his stuck points. He looked over the remaining chapters and realized that he felt pretty good about himself and others. He skipped ahead to the "Planning for the Conclusion of CPT" section and then to the final chapter to wrap up his work. He completed the final practice exercise by writing a Final Impact Statement about what he believes now about why the trauma happened and what his current beliefs are about himself, others, and the world. His Final Impact Statement was totally different from his first one because he no longer believed the stuck points he started with. Marcus decided that he didn't need to spend more time on it. He completed the program in six weeks.

Emily had been the victim of abuse as a child and was in a very abusive relationship as an adult. It took her several years to get to safety. By then she had sustained several concussions that left her with ringing ears and frequent headaches. Emily needed to read each chapter and watch the videos several times to understand and remember the concepts, and she practiced the worksheets repeatedly. She read them over to herself because sometimes she forgot what she had reasoned out before. Over time the headaches diminished but she understood that it would take a lot of practice to change her thinking patterns that had started in childhood and continued through the brutality of her partner, who reinforced the idea that she was worthless and unlovable. She spent three months going through the program daily and continues to use her worksheets occasionally.

Part IV

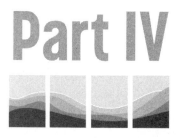

Getting Unstuck from Trauma-Related Beliefs about the Present and Future

Now that you've started using the Alternative Thoughts Worksheet (page 137) to examine your stuck points, you'll start to apply it to specific themes that often arise for people who experience PTSD. Don't worry if you're still practicing and getting the hang of the process. The important thing is to keep using the skills. You can also keep going back to your completed worksheets or rereading the material whenever you feel stuck. The Alternative Thoughts Worksheets will get easier as you practice with them. Remember that the worksheet is a tool for *you*. The goal isn't to fill it out "perfectly"—it's to use it to figure out a new belief that feels more balanced or accurate and that reduces your symptoms.

Themes That Can Be Disrupted by Traumatic Events

In addition to continuing to work on stuck points about the causes of traumatic events in your life, you can now begin to focus on the consequences of the traumatic events on your beliefs about yourself and others. In particular, you'll have the opportunity to examine five themes that are often disrupted by traumatic events:

safety, trust, power/control, esteem, and intimacy. We'll cover each of these topics one at a time in the next five chapters.

Each of these themes can be focused on yourself or outward toward others. Also, a focus across all five themes is identifying whether any of your thoughts are examples of all–or–none or either/or thinking (such as "I either trust you or I don't" or "I am completely safe or completely unsafe") and, if so, to develop realistic ways of looking at the situation based on all of the evidence and considering each theme on a continuum. For example, with esteem, do you have to be perfect in every way to be considered a worthwhile person? Can you have strengths and weaknesses? We also hope you'll recognize that, with each of these themes, there are different categories to consider. For example, whether you're thinking about safety, trust, power/control, esteem, or intimacy, you'll want to consider "What do I mean when I think about this topic?" "What kind of intimacy (sexual intimacy versus opening up to a friend about your emotions)?" "Control over what (control over biting your fingernails versus control over your child)?" Throughout, it will be helpful to think about how there are different types of safety, trust, power/control, esteem, and intimacy, and that they all fall on a continuum and are not just all–or–none.

We recommend going in the order that the chapters are presented in the book, even if you know that some themes are going to be more relevant for you than others. Sometimes working on those that come first can help you when you get to the next one.

11

Safety

The first theme that is often affected by trauma is safety. The fact that you (or someone else) were not safe when the traumatic event occurred may have led you to one of two conclusions: (1) if you thought that you would likely be safe in your day-to-day life before the trauma occurred, after the trauma you might have jumped to the opposite extreme, assuming that everywhere or everyone is dangerous; or (2) if you had prior experience with trauma or someone had already taught you that the world is dangerous, this trauma may have added to and strengthened that idea. However, as unsafe as the trauma left you feeling, in reality people are not in danger every minute of their lives and in every location. Your level of safety is different in different situations. Traumatic events happen occasionally or rarely, not usually daily. Of course, if you grew up in an abusive home or if you were in an abusive relationship, a threat was present whenever your abuser was around. But in many cases, the abuse is not constant, all day every day, and there are times of relative safety, like when the person who abused you was at work or asleep. Even in a country at war, there are locations that are more or less dangerous, and even in the dangerous parts of a city or country, violence does not usually occur constantly. Natural disasters may be generally predictable (such as hurricane season or brush fires in a dry summer), but many people and homes in the area are spared in natural disasters. Nonetheless, PTSD leaves people believing that they need to be on guard all the time, even at times when the threat level is actually fairly low, and this hypervigilance comes at a cost.

After a trauma, people's sense of the probability that something bad will happen (either experiencing the same trauma again or experiencing another trauma) is often affected. People often think the odds are quite high. But if you think there is a fifty–fifty chance of something bad happening when you leave your house or go to a certain place, that means you're thinking that you'll experience a trauma every other time you are in that situation. When you think of it that way, is it really fifty–fifty (meaning it would happen every other time)? Maybe think about someone you know who doesn't have the same safety concerns as you. Are they harmed every other time they go out or go somewhere crowded?

In CPT, we sometimes work with people to estimate the probability that something bad will happen based on the information they are able to access. Using real numbers often helps people see that, in many cases, the chance is much smaller than they thought. Dealing with safety means standing back and putting what happened to you in a larger context. How many times did you leave the house or drive on that road without having anything bad happen? How many parties have you attended where nothing bad happened during or afterward? How many hurricanes or tornadoes have occurred in your area over the past decade that have left your home and loved ones safe and intact? The fact that one time something bad did happen, while incredibly tragic, doesn't increase the overall odds that it will happen again. It's also possible that you might develop heightened attention to traumatic events in the news that you may have ignored before. Your perception of the probability that these events will occur is greater, not because the rates have gone up but because you are paying more attention to events that are similar to yours. In fact, if these events were very common, they would not report them in the news.

> Roberto was a veteran who experienced multiple combat traumas. Prior to developing PTSD, he enjoyed going to clubs and concerts to hear music with his wife. However, a few years ago he began to see more and more news stories about shootings at concerts. He formed the stuck points "It's not safe to go to concerts" and "If we go to a concert, we'll be shot." He had some evidence for these thoughts. The 2017 Las Vegas shooting was the deadliest mass shooting committed by an individual in U.S. history. Sixty people were killed, and 411 were wounded. The ensuing panic increased the number of people who were injured to 867. Roberto and his therapist looked closely at the numbers. Twenty-two thousand people had attended the concert. Roberto pulled out the calculator on his phone. If 60 out of 22,000 people were shot, that meant that if he had been at that concert, he would have had a risk of .0027 of being shot. That's less than a 1% chance even if he had been at the concert. Calculating the chance of being injured, he saw that there was about a 2% chance of being wounded directly from the shooting and about a 4% chance of being injured during the panic if he had been at the concert. Indeed, it was a terrifying experience for the people who were there.
>
> Roberto and his therapist thought about it more. How many other concerts were there all around the country that weekend where nothing like this had happened? How many concerts had there been since then where nothing had happened? In fact, there had been hundreds, with crowds ranging from a few hundred to several thousand. Thinking about it that way, Roberto realized that if he had gone to a concert somewhere in the United States on the weekend of the shooting in 2017, he had less than a one-in-a-million chance of being shot or injured. If he had gone to a concert the weekend before, he would have had a zero percent chance because he could find no news report of any shootings at concerts that spring weekend. Roberto then spent some time thinking about whether the very small risk of being at a concert where there was a shooting was worth giving up the enjoyment he and his wife had experienced for so many years when they went out to hear live music together.

It's important to remember that dangerous events do occur around the world, but how often do they happen to you, where you are?

How likely is it that on a specific day something bad will happen to you in the situation you are living in now? If you need to, check actual crime statistics for the area you live in or for a particular store or restaurant. Are you overestimating the likelihood of danger? If there was a crime or event, what was the nature of it? Was anyone physically harmed? If crimes occurred or people were harmed, how many people went to that place over the course of the past year and were unharmed or did not experience a trauma while they were there? How many times have you been there and *not* experienced a traumatic event? Write down what you conclude:

_____

_____

_____

_____

Now that you've thought about the probabilities of something bad happening in a place, activity, or situation you've been avoiding, *it's important to think about what it's costing you to live as though the probability of being harmed is very high.* There are costs in terms of our physical reactions, health, and also in terms of our quality of life.

First, let's think about the physical costs. Are you acting and feeling as though something bad is going to happen at any moment because triggers remind you of the event and you feel fear? Fight–flight–freeze reactions can help when we are in extreme danger, but not in small, everyday events. Research has shown that those reactions shut down your immune system and can lead to disease processes. People with untreated PTSD can have greater cardiac problems as well as other physical disorders. Therefore, it's important to learn when you are *not* in danger. Stop and think before you avoid, run, or fight. If no real danger is present, look around and notice if there was something that triggered an automatic thought and emotion. Do an Alternative Thoughts Worksheet (see pages 173–179) on the situation and stuck point as soon as possible. A possible stuck point may be "If there is any chance at all that it could happen again, I should always be on guard." You'll have to consider if that belief is realistic and if that's the way you want to live your life because of the physical consequences of anxiety and hypervigilance.

There are other costs to making decisions based on your judgments about safety. Some of these decisions end up maintaining or reinforcing your stuck points about safety. Avoidance and escape behaviors can be a real problem when it comes to safety stuck points. If you start to feel fear because of some reminder, your emotional reasoning might kick in and you might say to yourself, "I feel fear, so I must be in danger." You leave the situation and think that you've escaped from a dangerous situation (that may in fact have been perfectly safe). But because you escaped or avoided, you didn't learn that the situation was safe. Your thought might be "I just saved myself by running away" and your fear decreases temporarily. Your avoidance reinforces your stuck point, and your safety stuck points are unchanged or even increased.

As another example, if you tell yourself that "crowds are dangerous" and you avoid crowds, you never learn that many times crowds are not dangerous. You assume that by avoiding crowds you have just dodged danger. Like Roberto before he started CPT, you may not have noticed that nothing bad happened today to anyone at a sporting event or concert. You see the news on TV about something that happened somewhere else and say to yourself, "See, the world is too dangerous." You notice only what is on the news, but that's what makes it news, the fact that it's remarkable. The announcers on the news don't say how many thousands of events had nothing bad happen that day. That wouldn't be news, it would be usual. Millions of people fly safely every day, and they don't announce that on the news. The news broadcasts announce only the unusual situation, the one commercial airline crash out of millions of flights every year around the world. That particular crash doesn't make it more dangerous to fly—the statistics, the probabilities, haven't changed. It has just reminded you that things like that are *possible*. Experiencing a crime does not mean that the world is more dangerous. In fact, the crime rate may have gone down that year. It just happened that, unfortunately, you were one of the victims.

Another cost to making decisions based on overestimated risk is the cost to your quality of life. When you avoid situations that are generally safe, you might be giving up activities you used to enjoy. Have you gotten feedback from family or friends that they wish you would spend more time with them or that you would do things with them that you used to do? What is it costing them when you decide to keep avoiding? If you have children, what lessons are they learning about the world, and will they grow up learning to try new things?

Being aware of your surroundings is very different from being hypervigilant. Hypervigilance is actually bad for your health and won't prevent events. In fact, if you're always "on guard," it's harder to tell if you're in real danger because you come to distrust your own reactions. It's like setting the smoke detector in your house/apartment to such a sensitive level that every time you turn on the stove the alarm goes off and the fire truck comes. It's not actually making you safer. Instead, you can work on calibrating your alarm system. It can help to do worksheets on stuck points like "If I go out at night, I'll be assaulted" or "It's dangerous to go to parties" or whatever you notice saying to yourself about safety. When you are looking at evidence, you can get information about how safe or unsafe different activities or areas of town are.

In working on your worksheets, you may have begun to realize that being anxious or fearful and on guard does not prevent bad things from happening. If you had been afraid or not afraid, would the traumatic event have happened anyway? Part of recovery is working on focusing less on worries about future events and, instead, practicing standard caution and facing situations that are likely safe but that you have been avoiding. If there is no way to prevent the event, then your fear won't make any difference; it will happen whether or not you're afraid.

You can also figure out what standard precautions are by looking at what people around you who don't have PTSD do to be careful. For example, what do your colleagues who work the night shift with you do to take precautions without going overboard? A reasonable precaution might be to park near security, under a nearby streetlamp, or have someone walk you to your car if you need to park in a parking garage when you work late into the night.

It might be going overboard to always get a ride to work if there have been few or even no crimes reported in that parking garage over the past several months or years. What is it costing your friends or family in terms of, say, convenience, gas money, or lost sleep to give you a ride and pick you up every night? How will that help you begin to base your decisions on the facts around what's safe, rather than your stuck points?

Roberto kept working on his safety-related stuck points after he figured out the probabilities. The risk of being harmed if he went to a concert or a club to hear music wasn't zero, but it was lower than he thought. He began to think about what it was costing him to avoid these things. Not only was he not doing things he used to enjoy and noticing his mood was often lower as a result, but it was causing some problems with his family. His wife missed doing those things with him. It had been a way for them to connect around a shared interest and have some time together away from work and the kids. Now they rarely went out, and she felt sad and resentful about that.

Roberto had also seen how disappointed his daughter had been when he hadn't attended her dance performance. He had felt too anxious and had stuck points like "Something bad could happen in such a crowded place." So instead of watching her performance, he waited outside and watched the entrance to try to make sure nobody with a weapon entered the auditorium. But his daughter had noticed he wasn't there, and she felt very hurt by his absence.

His younger son was beginning to say that maybe it wasn't safe to play at the playground because he had heard Roberto talking about how unsafe the world was. Roberto realized that his fears were costing not only himself but also his family too much. He decided that avoiding the very small risk of harm was not worth giving up the kind of life that he and his family wanted to lead. He began gradually going back out to hear music with his wife, and he did a worksheet before his daughter's next performance, then went into the auditorium and watched the whole thing. He took his son to the playground and encouraged him to have fun. Roberto noticed how much better he felt and how much it meant to his family that he had begun to face his fears.

REFLECTION

What has it cost you and your loved ones to avoid things that started to feel less safe after your trauma? What have you given up? Are those costs worth limiting your activities and time with your loved ones? Has it prevented you from developing or keeping friendships?

_____

_____

_____

_____

It's also important, in thinking about safety, to think about self-safety. Since the traumatic event(s), have you decided that you are helpless or unable to protect yourself or reduce your risk for bad events happening? This kind of thinking can leave you anxious and withdrawn from others as well. It may lead you to be avoidant of any people or situations that you think could be dangerous because you doubt your ability to react appropriately to situations. Think back to the traumatic event. Were there some things that you did to help yourself or others during the event? It's possible that because only one image comes to mind when you remember the event, you have forgotten to look at the entire context of the event. If you are overly risk taking or overly cautious, you may have self-safety stuck points you need to think about.

☑ **Key Points about Safety**

Trauma can impact how you think about your own safety and how you think about whether and how safe you believe others and the world are.

Safety Beliefs Related to Self

Your sense of self-safety centers around the belief that you can protect yourself from harm and have some control over events. In response to traumatic events, you may become anxious, preoccupied with safety, or hypervigilant.

Your prior experiences may influence how you reacted to the trauma.

➲ If you grew up feeling safe and that you could protect yourself from harm, the traumatic event may have shaken up that belief.

➲ On the other hand, if you grew up in an unsafe environment where things felt dangerous and uncontrollable, you may have developed negative beliefs about your ability to stay safe and protect yourself. The traumatic event may have served to confirm those beliefs.

Below are some examples of how your beliefs might have changed, and some examples of new thoughts that might emerge as you carefully evaluate your own self-safety-related stuck points.

Pretrauma belief	Posttrauma stuck point	Possible balanced/alternative thought
I know how to protect myself.	I can't keep myself safe.	There are things I can do to protect myself even though there is no guarantee I'll be one hundred percent safe because I can't control everything that happens.

Pretrauma belief	Posttrauma stuck point	Possible balanced/alternative thought
I'm never safe.	I'll never be safe.	Some situations are safer than others, and there are some precautions I can take in many situations.
I'm generally safe.	It will happen to me again.	Something bad may happen again, but if I live my life every day like something bad is going to happen, I'll miss out on a lot of things I want to experience, and I'll be miserable.

Safety Beliefs Related to Others

Other-safety beliefs focus on whether other people are safe or dangerous and about whether the intent of others is to cause harm, hurt, or losses. You may become more isolated or withdrawn in response to trauma as a result of your experiences and beliefs. Or, you might be more angry and aggressive in defense.

Your prior experiences may also have shaped your response to the trauma.

➲ If you had experiences in which people were kind and safe to be around, you may have formed a belief that most people are safe and well intentioned. A traumatic event can shatter that belief.

➲ If you grew up in a dangerous environment or experienced or witnessed violence or danger regularly, other traumatic events you experience may seem to confirm the belief that other people are not safe to trust or be around or the world in general is dangerous.

Below are some examples of how your beliefs might have changed and some examples of new thoughts that might emerge as you carefully evaluate your other-safety-related stuck points.

Pretrauma belief	Posttrauma stuck point	Possible balanced/alternative thought
People are generally safe to be around and spend time with.	People are dangerous. You never know who will hurt you.	There may be some people who will harm others, but it is unrealistic to expect that everyone I meet will want to harm me.
Others are out to harm me.	I can never let my guard down.	It makes sense to take some precautions for people and situations I don't know, but there are people I can trust with my safety.

Pretrauma belief	Posttrauma stuck point	Possible balanced/alternative thought
The world is a safe place.	The world is dangerous. It's up to me to protect others.	Of course it makes sense to try to make sure my kids are in safe situations, but I also have to realize that I can't control every situation and that there are trade-offs to controlling situations so we all feel safe. I want my kids to have typical childhood experiences, and keeping them home or hovering over them will make that impossible.

▶▶ To watch a video to review what you just read about safety, go to the CPT White-board Video Library (*http://cptforptsd.com/cpt-resources*) and watch the video called *CPT Safety*.

 PRACTICE ASSIGNMENT

Look over your Stuck Point Log (page 56) to pick out the stuck points that are concerned with self- or other-safety. If you have issues with self- or other-safety, complete Alternative Thoughts Worksheets on them (see pages 173–179). Also notice whether you still have any stuck points related to safety about why the trauma happened—for example, "I should have been more on guard." If so, do those first.

With regard to safety stuck points, you need to include *all* of the evidence, not just facts or thoughts that support your stuck point. What are the **actual** probabilities that the event or something similar is going to happen again? Include all of the days before and since your trauma(s) in your perspective taking.

When you complete a worksheet that has a good alternative thought, read that work-sheet every day so that the new thought becomes your new habit.

Please complete the Alternative Thoughts Worksheets (pages 173–179) on your stuck points and focus particularly on safety stuck points.

 TROUBLESHOOTING

I'm still stuck. I'm having a hard time letting go of my safety beliefs.

If you're having a hard time letting go of your safety beliefs like "I must always be on guard," consider whether you still have any related *safety beliefs about why your traumatic event occurred*; if so, do those first. For example, if you're still thinking "The trauma happened because I wasn't on guard," or "If I had been more watchful, I could have prevented the trauma," it's

Alternative Thoughts Worksheet

A. Situation	B. Stuck point		D. Exploring thoughts	E. Thinking patterns	F. Alternative thought(s)
Describe the event leading to the stuck point or unpleasant emotion(s).	Write your stuck point related to the situation in Section A. Rate your belief in this stuck point from 0 to 100%. (How strongly do you believe this thought?)		Use the **exploring questions** to examine your automatic thought from Section B. Consider whether the thought is balanced and factual or extreme.	Use the **thinking patterns** to decide whether this is one of the patterns and explain why.	What else can you say instead of the thought in Section B? How else can you interpret the event instead of this thought? Rate your belief in the alternative thought(s) from 0 to 100%.
			Evidence against?	Jumping to conclusions:	
			What information is not included?	Ignoring important parts:	
			All or none? Extreme?		
			Focused on just one piece of the event?	Oversimplifying/overgeneralizing:	
	C. Emotion(s) Specify your emotion(s) (sad, angry, etc.) and rate how strongly you feel each emotion from 0 to 100%.		Questionable source of information?	Mind reading:	**G. Re-rate old stuck point** Re-rate how much you now believe the stuck point in Section B from 0 to 100%.
			Confusing possible with definite?		
			Based on feelings or facts?	Emotional reasoning:	**H. Emotion(s)** Now what do you feel? Rate from 0 to 100%.

Alternative Thoughts Worksheet

A. Situation	B. Stuck point	D. Exploring thoughts	E. Thinking patterns	F. Alternative thought(s)
Describe the event leading to the stuck point or unpleasant emotion(s).	Write your stuck point related to the situation in Section A. Rate your belief in this stuck point from 0 to 100%. (How strongly do you believe this thought?)	Use the **exploring questions** to examine your automatic thought from Section B. Consider whether the thought is balanced and factual or extreme.	Use the **thinking patterns** to decide whether this is one of the patterns and explain why.	What else can you say instead of the thought in Section B? How else can you interpret the event instead of this thought? Rate your belief in the alternative thought(s) from 0 to 100%.
		Evidence against?	Jumping to conclusions:	
		What information is not included?	Ignoring important parts:	
		All or none? Extreme?	Oversimplifying/overgeneralizing:	
	C. Emotion(s) Specify your emotion(s) (sad, angry, etc.) and rate how strongly you feel each emotion from 0 to 100%.	Focused on just one piece of the event?		**G. Re-rate old stuck point** Re-rate how much you now believe the stuck point in Section B from 0 to 100%.
		Questionable source of information?	Mind reading:	
		Confusing possible with definite?		
		Based on feelings or facts?	Emotional reasoning:	**H. Emotion(s)** Now what do you feel? Rate from 0 to 100%.

Alternative Thoughts Worksheet

A. Situation	B. Stuck point	C. Emotion(s)	D. Exploring thoughts	E. Thinking patterns	F. Alternative thought(s)	G. Re-rate old stuck point	H. Emotion(s)
Describe the event leading to the stuck point or unpleasant emotion(s).	Write your stuck point related to the situation in Section A. Rate your belief in this stuck point from 0 to 100%. (How strongly do you believe this thought?)	Specify your emotion(s) (sad, angry, etc.) and rate how strongly you feel each emotion from 0 to 100%.	Use the **exploring questions** to examine your automatic thought from Section B. Consider whether the thought is balanced and factual or extreme.	Use the **thinking patterns** to decide whether this is one of the patterns and explain why.	What else can you say instead of the thought in Section B? How else can you interpret the event instead of this thought? Rate your belief in the alternative thought(s) from 0 to 100%.	Re-rate how much you now believe the stuck point in Section B from 0 to 100%.	Now what do you feel? Rate from 0 to 100%.
			Evidence against?	Jumping to conclusions:			
			What information is not included?	Ignoring important parts:			
			All or none? Extreme?	Oversimplifying/overgeneralizing:			
			Focused on just one piece of the event?	Mind reading:			
			Questionable source of information?				
			Confusing possible with definite?	Emotional reasoning:			
			Based on feelings or facts?				

Alternative Thoughts Worksheet

A. Situation	B. Stuck point	C. Emotion(s)	D. Exploring thoughts	E. Thinking patterns	F. Alternative thought(s)
Describe the event leading to the stuck point or unpleasant emotion(s).	Write your stuck point related to the situation in Section A. Rate your belief in this stuck point from 0 to 100%. (How strongly do you believe this thought?)	Specify your emotion(s) (sad, angry, etc.) and rate how strongly you feel each emotion from 0 to 100%.	Use the **exploring questions** to examine your automatic thought from Section B. Consider whether the thought is balanced and factual or extreme.	Use the **thinking patterns** to decide whether this is one of the patterns and explain why.	What else can you say instead of the thought in Section B? How else can you interpret the event instead of this thought? Rate your belief in the alternative thought(s) from 0 to 100%.
			Evidence against?	Jumping to conclusions:	
			What information is not included?	Ignoring important parts:	
			All or none? Extreme?		
			Focused on just one piece of the event?	Oversimplifying/overgeneralizing:	
			Questionable source of information?	Mind reading:	**G. Re-rate old stuck point** Re-rate how much you now believe the stuck point in Section B from 0 to 100%.
			Confusing possible with definite?		
			Based on feelings or facts?	Emotional reasoning:	**H. Emotion(s)** Now what do you feel? Rate from 0 to 100%.

Alternative Thoughts Worksheet

A. Situation	B. Stuck point	D. Exploring thoughts	E. Thinking patterns	F. Alternative thought(s)
Describe the event leading to the stuck point or unpleasant emotion(s).	Write your stuck point related to the situation in Section A. Rate your belief in this stuck point from 0 to 100%. (How strongly do you believe this thought?)	Use the **exploring questions** to examine your automatic thought from Section B. Consider whether the thought is balanced and factual or extreme.	Use the **thinking patterns** to decide whether this is one of the patterns and explain why.	What else can you say instead of the thought in Section B? How else can you interpret the event instead of this thought? Rate your belief in the alternative thought(s) from 0 to 100%.
		Evidence against?	Jumping to conclusions:	
		What information is not included?	Ignoring important parts:	
		All or none? Extreme?		
		Focused on just one piece of the event?	Oversimplifying/overgeneralizing:	
	C. Emotion(s) Specify your emotion(s) (sad, angry, etc.) and rate how strongly you feel each emotion from 0 to 100%.	Questionable source of information?	Mind reading:	**G. Re-rate old stuck point** Re-rate how much you now believe the stuck point in Section B from 0 to 100%.
		Confusing possible with definite?		
		Based on feelings or facts?	Emotional reasoning:	**H. Emotion(s)** Now what do you feel? Rate from 0 to 100%.

Alternative Thoughts Worksheet

A. Situation	B. Stuck point	D. Exploring thoughts	E. Thinking patterns	F. Alternative thought(s)
Describe the event leading to the stuck point or unpleasant emotion(s).	Write your stuck point related to the situation in Section A. Rate your belief in this stuck point from 0 to 100%. (How strongly do you believe this thought?)	Use the **exploring questions** to examine your automatic thought from Section B. Consider whether the thought is balanced and factual or extreme.	Use the **thinking patterns** to decide whether this is one of the patterns and explain why.	What else can you say instead of the thought in Section B? How else can you interpret the event instead of this thought? Rate your belief in the alternative thought(s) from 0 to 100%.
		Evidence against?	Jumping to conclusions:	
		What information is not included?	Ignoring important parts:	
		All or none? Extreme?		
		Focused on just one piece of the event?	Oversimplifying/overgeneralizing:	
	C. Emotion(s) Specify your emotion(s) (sad, angry, etc.) and rate how strongly you feel each emotion from 0 to 100%.	Questionable source of information?	Mind reading:	**G. Re-rate old stuck point** Re-rate how much you now believe the stuck point in Section B from 0 to 100%.
		Confusing possible with definite?		
		Based on feelings or facts?	Emotional reasoning:	**H. Emotion(s)** Now what do you feel? Rate from 0 to 100%.

Alternative Thoughts Worksheet

A. Situation	B. Stuck point	C. Emotion(s)	D. Exploring thoughts	E. Thinking patterns	F. Alternative thought(s)
Describe the event leading to the stuck point or unpleasant emotion(s).	Write your stuck point related to the situation in Section A. Rate your belief in this stuck point from 0 to 100%. (How strongly do you believe this thought?)		Use the **exploring questions** to examine your automatic thought from Section B. Consider whether the thought is balanced and factual or extreme.	Use the **thinking patterns** to decide whether this is one of the patterns and explain why.	What else can you say instead of the thought in Section B? How else can you interpret the event instead of this thought? Rate your belief in the alternative thought(s) from 0 to 100%.
			Evidence against?	Jumping to conclusions:	
			What information is not included?	Ignoring important parts:	
			All or none? Extreme?	Oversimplifying/overgeneralizing:	
			Focused on just one piece of the event?		
		C. Emotion(s) Specify your emotion(s) (sad, angry, etc.) and rate how strongly you feel each emotion from 0 to 100%.	Questionable source of information?	Mind reading:	**G. Re-rate old stuck point** Re-rate how much you now believe the stuck point in Section B from 0 to 100%.
			Confusing possible with definite?		
			Based on feelings or facts?	Emotional reasoning:	**H. Emotion(s)** Now what do you feel? Rate from 0 to 100%.

From *Getting Unstuck from PTSD* by Patricia A. Resick, Shannon Wiltsey Stirman, and Stefanie T. LoSavio. Copyright © 2023 The Guilford Press. Purchasers of this book can photocopy and/or download additional copies of this worksheet at *www.guilford.com/resick2-forms* for personal use or use with clients; see copyright page for details.

no surprise that you still think it's important to be on guard at all times. However, reconsider the facts of the trauma. Did the trauma happen because you weren't on guard, or was it because of something out of your control, like because of an accident or because someone decided to hurt you? Can all events be prevented? Go back and do an Alternative Thoughts Worksheet on the safety stuck point about why the trauma happened. Then see if you can make progress on the more general stuck points about safety in your everyday life.

If you grew up in a dangerous environment with frequent violence, safety beliefs may have become core beliefs. You may not even think about dangerousness anymore but just assume that everyone and everyplace is dangerous. If this is a core belief, you may need to do many worksheets before you start to loosen the grip on those assumptions.

Even if there is one chance in a million, I don't want to take it.

It's understandable that if you've experienced trauma, you never want to experience anything like that again. It's your choice if you want to continue your safety behaviors like hypervigilance, but it's important to consider how doing so affects your ability to move toward your goals. We all face risks when we don't know what's going to happen in the future. But what is the quality of your life now, and how might it be if you were able to engage in some low-risk activities? Also, is there a stuck point behind that statement that indicates you think you couldn't tolerate something bad happening to you in the future? Unfortunately, there are no guarantees that a bad thing won't happen, even if you isolate yourself or stay home all the time. And what have you sacrificed in order to try to protect yourself from any negative outcomes?

I understand logically that the chances are low, but I still feel scared.

It makes sense to feel some degree of fear acknowledging the fact that the risk of something happening is never zero. That being said, remember our old enemy: avoidance. If your habit had been to run away when you felt fear, it might be emotional reasoning and you haven't had a chance to learn that in many situations you may actually not have experienced harm if you had stayed. If you face safe but avoided situations, fear will reduce eventually as you allow yourself to experience them.

What if I do live in a dangerous neighborhood/situation?

It's important to recognize that some places and situations really are less safe than others. However, if you're in a less safe place or situation, take a close look. Is the danger at a constant level, twenty-four hours a day? Or are there times that are more or less dangerous? Even in war zones, there are areas and times of day that are more or less dangerous. In the meantime, there is a difference between being cautious and being hypervigilant. Look at or talk to the neighbors who haven't had problems in the neighborhood and see what they feel comfortable doing and what precautions they take. How dangerous do they think the neighborhood is? Are there things within your control that could make your home or work safer?

If you are living in a dangerous situation, like in a situation where there is domestic violence, there may be agencies that can help you. If you have access to support or resources to work toward living in a safer environment, it might be useful to come up with a plan, even if it needs to be a longer-term plan. Do you have family or friends who can help? You may need to develop a safety plan so that you can get out of the house with what you need all ready and a safe place to go. If you need outside help and you live in the United States, consider contacting the National Domestic Violence Hotline at *www.thehotline.org*. You can call them at 1-800-799-SAFE (7233) or TTY 1-800-787-3224. You can also chat live or text from the website. They provide instructions about how to keep your conversation safe.

*   *   *

Continue to track your progress by completing the PTSD Checklist again and using the Graph for Tracking Your Weekly Scores found on page 24. Remember that when your score gets below 20, you may want to assess whether you have worked on all of the stuck points you need to and are ready to move toward wrapping up. Whenever you're ready, you can go to the section called "Planning for the Conclusion of CPT" on page 264. Otherwise, keep working on your stuck points. If you feel stuck, refer back to the section called "If You Are Not Noticing Change" in the "Reflecting on Your Progress" part of the book (pages 152–156) and reread earlier sections of the book as needed.

(PTSD Checklist)

Complete the PTSD Checklist to track your symptoms as you complete this book. Be sure to complete this measure on the same index event each time. When the instructions and questions refer to a "stressful experience," remember that that is your index event—the worst event that you are working on first.

Write in here the trauma that you are working on first: _____

Complete this PTSD Checklist with reference to that event.

Instructions: Below is a list of problems that people sometimes have in response to a very stressful experience. Please read each problem carefully, and then circle one of the numbers to the right to indicate how much you have been bothered by that problem *in the past week*.

In the past week, how much were you bothered by:	Not at all	A little bit	Mod- erately	Quite a bit	Extremely
1. Repeated, disturbing, and unwanted memories of the stressful experience?	0	1	2	3	4
2. Repeated, disturbing dreams of the stressful experience?	0	1	2	3	4
3. Suddenly feeling or acting as if the stressful experience were actually happening again (*as if you were actually back there reliving it*)?	0	1	2	3	4
4. Feeling very upset when something reminded you of the stressful experience?	0	1	2	3	4
5. Having strong physical reactions when something reminded you of the stressful experience (*for example, heart pounding, trouble breathing, sweating*)?	0	1	2	3	4
6. Avoiding memories, thoughts, or feelings related to the stressful experience?	0	1	2	3	4
7. Avoiding external reminders of the stressful experience (*for example, people, places, conversations, activities, objects, or situations*)?	0	1	2	3	4
8. Trouble remembering important parts of the stressful experience (not due to head injury or substances)?	0	1	2	3	4
9. Having strong negative beliefs about yourself, other people, or the world (*for example, having thoughts such as I am bad, There is something seriously wrong with me, No one can be trusted, or The world is completely dangerous*)?	0	1	2	3	4
10. Blaming yourself or someone else (who didn't intend the outcome) for the stressful experience or what happened after it?	0	1	2	3	4
11. Having strong negative feelings, such as fear, horror, anger, guilt, or shame?	0	1	2	3	4
12. Loss of interest in activities that you used to enjoy?	0	1	2	3	4
13. Feeling distant or cut off from other people?	0	1	2	3	4
14. Trouble experiencing positive feelings (*for example, being unable to feel happiness or have loving feelings for people close to you*)?	0	1	2	3	4
15. Irritable behavior, angry outbursts, or acting aggressively?	0	1	2	3	4
16. Taking too many risks or doing things that could cause you harm?	0	1	2	3	4
17. Being "super alert" or watchful or on guard?	0	1	2	3	4
18. Feeling jumpy or easily startled?	0	1	2	3	4
19. Having difficulty concentrating?	0	1	2	3	4
20. Trouble falling or staying asleep?	0	1	2	3	4

Add up the total and write it here: _____

12

Trust

Traumatic events can have a profound impact on your sense of trust. If you grew up believing that others are basically trustworthy, you may notice that the trauma turned that belief upside down, and you might have formed a stuck point like "I can't trust anyone." Especially if someone you trusted hurt or betrayed you, you may have also developed different beliefs about whether you can trust yourself or your own judgment. Just as you probably need to work on resetting the sensitivity of your alarm when it comes to safety, you may need to recalibrate your sense of trust.

One of the biggest problems, though, is that the word *trust* is too vague and too big. What do you mean by trust? When you think about trust currently, you may be thinking about trust only with regard to your life or trust that someone won't betray you. But there are many kinds of trust, and it's impossible to trust people in every possible way. However, that doesn't mean that you should not trust someone at all. The trick is to figure out in which *ways* you trust someone and *how much* you want to let them into your life in that way.

You may think there are only two options, trust and not trust. Sometimes it's only necessary to trust someone in one kind of way. For example, the person who cuts your hair does that well, so you trust them to do it, but you might not trust them with a secret or that they'll pay you back if you loan them money, because that may not matter for the type of relationship you have with them. Trust is also not all-or-none but falls along a continuum from a little bit to a great deal. For a lot of things, you may not actually have enough information to know if you can trust someone in some particular way. There may be things you don't know because you haven't had the opportunity to find out. You may need to get to know the person more to find out how trustworthy they are in that way, or you may never need to know, depending on the kind of relationship you have with them.

There are many different kinds of trust. Following are just a few examples, though there are many more.

Examples of Kinds of Trust

- Keeping a secret
- Not using information about you to hurt you

- Being on time (or for some people, you can trust that they will always be late!)
- Loaning someone money and getting it back
- That you can talk to someone when you have a problem
- That your doctor will take care of your health
- That your mechanic will fix your car
- That your partner will be faithful to you
- Being reliable; someone does what they say they are going to do
- Taking care of your children or pets well
- Trusting your own judgment or decision making

What other kinds of trust can you think of that are important to you?

_____

_____

_____

_____

The Trust Star

The purpose of the Trust Star Worksheet (page 187) is to think about trust not so much as an all-or-none ("I either trust you or I don't") but to consider **to what degree you trust someone and with what.** You can work on trust stars to think through your trust for yourself or someone else you trust in at least some ways. Following are instructions:

1. List all of the different kinds of trust you can think of. You can use the kinds of trust listed above and on the previous page or any that you have thought of since then. Try to think of some that especially apply to the person you want to rate.

2. Put a star by three or four items that are most important to you and start with them on the Trust Star Worksheet on page 187. You can also download and print the Trust Star Worksheet from *www.guilford.com/resick2-forms*.

3. Pick a person in your life who you think might be trustworthy in at least some areas. Maybe there is someone you know you can trust to drive safely and take care of your children, pets, or property, or someone you know you can talk with about how you are feeling.

4. Each line on the star represents a type of trust. You'll notice that the lines have a scale from "−" to "+" to indicate how much you trust a person in each area. If you trust the person completely in one way, put an "X" out at the end of the line with the

+ sign. If you trust them partially, put the X along the line for approximately how much you trust them. For example, if someone is not reliable in a particular way, you might rate them on the side with the minus sign. If you don't have any information about whether you can trust that person in that specific area, put the X in the middle section, indicating **no information**. Next, do that with other kinds of trust.

5. Now look at how you have assessed this person. Can you mostly trust them with the important kinds of trust? If so, that's someone you might want to stay close to or develop a deeper relationship with. If the person is mostly on the negative side, this is someone you may not want to have in your life very much or with whom to limit your contact to more superficial activities.

A filled-in example of the Trust Star Worksheet can be found on the next page, and a blank version for your use is on page 187.

> ⏩ To watch a video to review what you just read about the Trust Star, go to the CPT Whiteboard Video Library (*http://cptforptsd.com/cpt-resources*) and watch the video called *Trust I: How Do I Know If I Can Trust Someone?*

Iryna completed the Trust Star using her friend since childhood, Tamara, as an example. She observed that her friend was particularly trustworthy in the areas of providing emotional support and keeping her safe. Their whole lives, Tamara had demonstrated a pattern of looking out for Iryna and showing her respect and kindness. When Iryna had her daughter, Tamara was often helpful and sometimes watched her while Iryna worked. Nevertheless, even a supportive and helpful friend like Tamara wasn't a perfect person. Iryna noted that Tamara often ran behind schedule due to being a daydreamer and getting absorbed in conversations and books. Although she would always show up, sometimes she would be up to an hour late. Earlier in their relationship, sometimes this behavior annoyed Iryna, and she once confronted Tamara about it when she was supposed to watch Iryna's daughter and Iryna ended up being late to an important meeting at work. Tamara apologized, and Iryna knew she was sincere, but Tamara would still run late occasionally. Iryna came to understand this fact about her friend and just made accommodations so that if Tamara was not on time, Iryna wouldn't be dependent on her arrival. Iryna also reflected that there were some types of trust that had just never been part of their relationship. For example, Iryna had never lent Tamara money, so she had no idea whether Tamara would be good at remembering to repay money. Because this wasn't part of their relationship, it wasn't an important kind of trust to consider. However, Iryna felt confident she would continue to lean on Tamara for emotional support and feel confident leaving her daughter in her care. In fact, these kinds of trust were the most important to Iryna.

Example Trust Star Worksheet

There are many different types of trust (for example, keeping secrets, being reliable). In the blanks below, list all the different types of trust you can think of. Then think about one particular person. Write in your relationship with them here: _childhood friend_. If you cannot think of a family member or friend, think of someone in whom you must place your trust, like a doctor, mechanic, or bus driver. Put a star by the most important types of trust for that person. Then fill in the star by writing a type of trust on the line along the star and putting an "X" on the line indicating how much you trust them with that type of trust. If you don't know, put the "X" just inside the "no information" circle (for example, "Returns money" below). Does this person need to be trustworthy in *every* way? What about the most important ways? Would you trust this person to pull your tooth, cut your hair, fix your car?

Types of Trust

Keeps private information*	Trust with my child*	Returns money
Reliable	On time	Supportive*
Protective*	Competent	Faithful
Doesn't gossip	Keep me physically safe*	

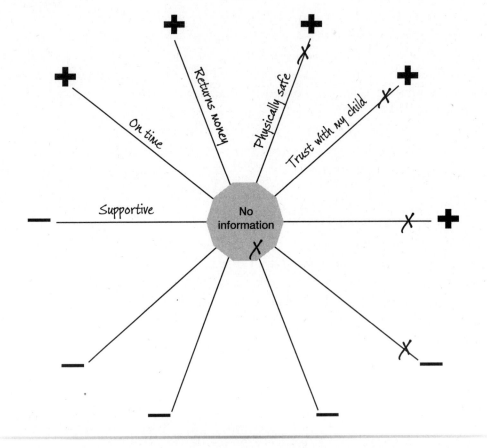

There are many different types of trust (for example, keeping secrets, being reliable). In the blanks below, list all the different types of trust you can think of. Then think about one particular person. Write in your relationship with them here: _____. If you cannot think of a family member or friend, think of someone in whom you must place your trust, like a doctor, mechanic, or bus driver. Put a star by the most important types of trust for that person. Then fill in the star by writing a type of trust on the line along the star and putting an "X" on the line indicating how much you trust them with that type of trust. If you don't know, put the "X" just inside the "no information" circle. Does this person need to be trustworthy in *every* way? What about the most important ways? Would you trust this person to pull your tooth, cut your hair, fix your car?

Types of Trust

_____   _____   _____

_____   _____   _____

_____   _____   _____

_____   _____   _____

No information

What did you take away from the Trust Star Worksheet?

_____

_____

_____

_____

Takeaways about Trust

• Trust is not one thing. There are many different ways to trust (for example, trusting someone to tell the truth, be supportive when you share personal information, be on time, pay back money, care for your pets).

• Trust is not all-or-none. It's on a continuum, a scale.

• We find out how trustworthy someone is with something through experience. Based on their actions, we might decide to trust them more or less on that type of trust.

• It helps to start small. If you want to find out how trustworthy someone is with paying back money, you might start by lending them five dollars, not a hundred dollars. Over time, you may be more willing to lend larger amounts if they have proven themselves trustworthy with paying you back.

• We want to start out assuming we have no information about someone. They are neither completely trustworthy nor completely untrustworthy until we learn more. Trusting someone completely before having much experience with them can lead to disappointments. On the other hand, keeping people at a distance without ever giving them a chance, or "testing" them repeatedly, might lead to missing out on good relationships.

• You might have certain trust deal breakers, but, generally speaking, if someone lets you down in an area, you might consider sharing with them how their actions affected you and asking for change. Those who change willingly are exactly the kinds of people we want in our lives. However, if they don't change, it isn't wise to keep trusting them in that area.

• People can be more trustworthy in some areas than others, and that doesn't mean you need to write them off. You can be thoughtful about what you trust them with.

Please note: The Trust Star can be used for any of the five themes covered in this book: safety, trust, power/control, esteem, and intimacy. All of these topics involve thinking about different categories and considering them on a continuum (for example, different kinds and degrees of intimacy).

Building Trust

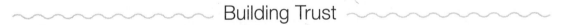

Now that you've done this exercise, you can see that there are some ways in which you trust people in your life more than others. You can make decisions about how much to trust them based on this more balanced view, instead of making an all-or-none decision. If you find yourself not knowing much about a person, there are other ways to obtain information about them. It makes sense to take things slowly and learn more about them before making decisions about how much to trust them. A balanced approach to trusting someone new is to begin by being fairly neutral: not to trust them completely right away, but also not to decide immediately that you don't trust them (start from a no-information position). We learn through our experiences, and you won't have any experience with someone you just met. You can also watch people and see how they behave with the other people in their lives. Do they blab secrets or gossip about them? Do they show other people respect? Do they show up on time or fulfill their responsibilities and obligations? What do other people say about them?

You can also take a small risk by trusting someone with something small—perhaps loaning them a small amount of money if they ask (for example, if they accidentally left their wallet at home and ask to borrow ten dollars for lunch) or telling them something that doesn't feel too personal about yourself and seeing how they react or whether they tell others, rather than immediately telling them about your trauma history. Over time, you may decide you can trust them more or less in different areas based on your experiences with them.

Starting at "No Information"

Many people we have worked with have told us that they start out assuming people are completely untrustworthy. If someone new comes into their life or is interested in being their friend or dating them, they put up walls and may put people to the test and make them prove themselves over and over again before giving these new people in their lives a real chance. One problem with this approach is that it might weed out some really great people with whom you might be able to have a fulfilling relationship. Someone who is really respectful of other people will not stick around and play games because if you say, "No, I don't trust you," they will say, "OK, I understand. I will leave you alone." In other words, people who respect other people's boundaries won't push you, and so you might not get a chance to know them if your walls are built too high. On the other hand, some people may push you to drop your guard, seemingly earning your trust by giving you lots of attention and being very persistent. These people may or may not turn out to be the kind of people you want to have in your life. So work on assuming "I have no information about this person yet" and neither trusting or not trusting them yet.

Second Chances

As you work on building trust, remember that people are not perfect. Just as you may want or need a second chance from people in your life when you make a mistake, you may find that it's important to give others a second chance in some circumstances. Sometimes people make mistakes and may hurt your feelings or let you down in some way. They may not even realize that they have done that. If you don't like how someone has behaved, tell them so assertively, but not aggressively. It may take time for you to rebuild trust with them through consistent action that shows that they can be trusted again, especially if they have violated your trust in a fundamental way, such as through marital infidelity or financial exploitation. You can make choices about whether their efforts to change are sufficient to feel comfortable trusting them in these areas again. If they have harmed you in a way that you decide is unforgivable, or there is evidence that trusting them again is not in your best interest, you can decide to have little or nothing to do with them from now on. However, in some relationships you may decide to limit future trust to only certain areas, based on evidence you see on their trustworthiness in those individual areas.

Rebuilding Trust After a Mistake

Let's look at an example where someone betrays your trust by telling someone else a secret that you told them. How can you handle that in a way that gives them a chance to rebuild trust without taking too big a risk? First, remember that they may not have known that something you told them was confidential if you didn't tell them not to discuss it with others. They may have assumed that, since you told them, you were open about this information. Whether or not they knew, you can say something like, "When you told what I shared with you, I felt betrayed. Please don't do that again. I will also make sure to tell you when something is just between us." If they apologize and say they won't do it again, you can work on slowly rebuilding trust by not telling them things that are big secrets until they have been trustworthy with your smaller secrets. If they don't violate your trust again, they may very well be someone you want to keep in your life. They have changed for you and shown you that they want to, and can be, trustworthy for you. By following this process, you'll eventually learn who you might want to have a casual friendship with, just talk to occasionally, spend more time with, go out of your way to help, or trust with confidential information.

> Maria immigrated to the United States with her family when she was twelve years old. She was targeted for being different from her classmates, and some kids even physically touched and threatened her. She didn't believe people in authority cared about or would help her, ever since the principal refused to punish kids at school for making fun of her accent and grabbing her breasts on the playground, and a teacher had singled her out and mocked her with slurs and stereotypes about her culture. As a result, she was very guarded and slow to form friendships. When she was in high school, Maria witnessed her brother being beaten and almost killed in a hate crime, and when police arrived at the scene, they were slow to intervene because the father of one of the perpetrators was a prominent politician in the small town. After that, she quit jobs abruptly throughout high school because she feared that her bosses would not have her back if customers called her disrespectful names. She also believed she couldn't trust anyone she met because she had seen how her classmates became increasingly abusive toward her and her brother as they got older. As a result, she had very few friends.

When Maria moved away from home, she began dating and making friends with people from similar backgrounds as her, though, she would jump into relationships very quickly, sharing a lot about herself and her past before she really knew her partner well. She assumed that they would understand her and protect her feelings because they understood what it was like to have experiences like hers. However, some partners pulled away or abruptly ended the relationship, which reinforced her belief that she couldn't really trust anyone to take care of her feelings. As she examined her stuck points about trust, she began to recognize that assuming she could trust people one hundred percent with her secrets and feelings was no healthier than assuming she couldn't trust anyone at all. She began to share things about herself more gradually and paid attention to how people reacted. She used their reactions as evidence on her worksheets about trust. She made lists going from low-cost/low-vulnerability information to share to higher-vulnerability information to share (like disclosing her brother's assault and difficult memories about her childhood).

Maria decided what kinds of reactions she would need to see from people to share more information as she began to disclose more moderately difficult memories and details about her life. That way she was able to use the information she was gathering to decide whether to share more or to get closer to people. As she got into a romantic relationship, she also told her partner when things they said hurt her feelings or hit a nerve, and she asked them to be more considerate. Her partner reacted positively and adjusted their behavior. Over time they developed a healthy and connected relationship.

Don't assume that you had to have known the perpetrator to have trust issues with others. We have heard many people say of assaults by strangers, "That means I can't trust anyone." Of course, the questions that a therapist might ask are "What does an attack by a stranger have to do with trust? Did you have to trust the stranger for the person to hurt you?"

Trusting People with Information about Your Trauma and PTSD

It's important to know that you are under no obligation to share information or details about your trauma with anyone you don't feel comfortable sharing that information with. In fact, it may be better to choose carefully whom you tell, and what level of detail you share, because not everyone knows how, or is willing, to be supportive (especially if they have a tendency to blame you because of their own just-world beliefs). You may choose not to say anything to some people. If others need to know something (for example, if your employer needs to know that you go to therapy), you might just share that you experienced a trauma and leave it at that. Still others might be supportive or might be able to relate, and you might find it safe to discuss what happened in more detail. But you can be the one who decides that. By gradually sharing information with people who seem supportive or understanding, you may find the people who can ultimately be trusted with more of your feelings and memories and who are able to support you.

If you find that people aren't helpful or supportive in their responses to that information, you can give them feedback. You can adjust how much you share or spend time with them based on how they react to that feedback. Some people may believe so strongly in the just-world belief that they may continue to be blaming and unsupportive. It's OK to distance yourself from them. Others may not be able or may not know how to support you, and they may not be very helpful but are kind or enjoyable to spend time with in other ways. In these cases, you may choose to limit your interactions with them to activities and topics that feel emotionally safer.

☑ **Key Points about Trust**

Trust Beliefs Related to Self

Self-related beliefs center around how much you believe you can trust or rely on your own perceptions or judgments. The ability to trust yourself is key to your sense of self, and it can help you protect yourself from doing things that don't feel right to you or being taken advantage of or emotionally hurt.

Your prior experiences also shaped your sense of trust after the trauma.

➲ If you grew up believing that you had good judgment and trusting your instincts and assessment of people and situations, the trauma may have turned that belief upside down.

➲ On the other hand, if you were often blamed when things went wrong, or if you were hurt by people you trusted, you may have begun to believe you can't make good decisions and that you aren't a good judge of character. The trauma may have confirmed that belief in your mind.

As a result of these patterns, you may find yourself to be anxious and full of self-doubt or criticism and you may often feel indecisive. You might feel a big sense of betrayal over things that others might not be as bothered by, like someone canceling plans or being late.

Pretrauma belief	Posttrauma stuck point	Possible balanced/alternative thought
I can trust myself to make good decisions.	I make bad decisions. I should never trust my instincts.	I couldn't have predicted what would happen based on the information I had. I did the best I could in an unpredictable situation.
		People can make mistakes but still have good judgment. In fact, everyone makes mistakes sometimes. Even when I do make mistakes, it doesn't mean I can't trust myself at all.

Pretrauma belief	Posttrauma stuck point	Possible balanced/alternative thought
I'm a terrible judge of character/ I make bad decisions.	I can't trust myself at all.	I made the best decisions I could with the information I had. I can't always know everything about how things will turn out, and I can't always predict what other people will do. I may have started doubting myself because of messages I got from others when I was young, but when I step back and look at it, I get it right sometimes and I make better decisions than I give myself credit for.
I can trust my instincts	I always have to trust my gut or I'll get hurt.	Sometimes a person or situation might really be "off." I can use the CPT skills I've learned to figure out whether it's a false alarm and to decide when to trust those feelings.

Trust Beliefs Related to Others

Trust is the belief that the promises of other people or groups can be relied on in terms of future behavior. We begin to learn to trust or mistrust others very early in life. Over time, ideally people learn a healthy balance of trust and mistrust and when it's appropriate to trust others or to be wary.

- ⮑ If you had good experiences with people growing up, you may have come to believe that all or most people can be trusted. The traumatic event may make you doubt that.

- ⮑ If you experienced betrayal or neglect earlier in life, you may have come to believe that you can't trust anyone. The trauma may have seemed to confirm that, especially if you were harmed by someone you knew.

If, after traumatic events, people you trusted were blaming, critical, or distant (perhaps because they didn't know what to say or how to help you) or unsupportive in some way, you may have felt disillusioned, angry, or betrayed, and you may have concluded that even people you thought were trustworthy can't be trusted.

As a result of the patterns you experience, you may find yourself to be extremely cautious. You may feel angry and suspicious about others' behaviors. You may find yourself avoiding close relationships or believing that something seemingly small is proof that you can't really trust someone. You might find that you are often afraid of being betrayed.

Pretrauma belief	Posttrauma stuck point	Possible balanced/alternative thought
I can trust my friends and my family.	Sooner or later, everyone betrays you.	Some people might let me down, but that doesn't mean that I can't trust the people I used to trust. Even if someone lets me down in some way, I can tell them how they hurt me and give them another chance. That's what I would want if I let someone who I care about down.
People are generally trustworthy.	Nobody can be trusted.	Some may be more trustworthy than others, and I may be able to trust some people with things like money, or helping with my kids, but not other things, like secrets. I can see how people respond to feedback and reasonable requests and decide how much to interact with them.
Watch your back. People can't be trusted.	If someone hurts me, it's my fault for trusting.	Trust involves some risk, but I can protect myself by developing trust slowly and basing it on what I learn about that person as I get to know them. I can't completely predict what people will do, but the cost of not trusting anyone at all is being lonely and isolated.

Betrayal of Trust

Whether about the trauma or related to other relationships you have had, many people assume that their trusting the other person was the reason they had a bad outcome. It may be helpful to ask yourself questions like the following: Why did you initially trust that person? Was it obvious then that they were going to be harmful to you, or did they seem trustworthy at the time? Many people we have worked with have told us that a person who eventually abused them initially was kind to them and made them feel special. They may have given you a lot of their attention and promised to be good to you. When you remember how the person initially treated you, does it make sense that you trusted them? Might it even say something good about you that you were open and gave someone a chance?

Sometimes people look back after the fact, in hindsight, and say to themselves, "I should have seen the signs." For example, they look back and see that someone who eventually became an abuser was controlling or sometimes put them down. If that was the case, what did you think at the time? Did you think it would lead to what it did (for example, physical or sexual violence)? What were you hoping? Did they apologize and say they would do better? Did you hope that they would go to counseling and that the relationship would improve? Did that person tell you that you were the only one who could help them? If so, does it make sense that you gave them another chance? And if they had actually done better and started treating you better, would you be going back and beating yourself up for giving them another chance?

Also, sometimes people look back and remember having an uneasy feeling about someone. Some people say they had a "gut feeling" or "instinct" that they ignored. Even if you had a feeling, did the feeling tell you exactly what to do and when? Have you ever had a bad feeling but everything turned out fine? Even if you had a feeling, was there a reason you didn't listen to it? For example, did you have prior experiences that made you question your own feelings and judgment?

Finally, sometimes people look back and see that many people have hurt them and assume it must be because of them. In fact, it's actually quite common for people to be revictimized in the course of their life. Sometimes people even prey on people who have been hurt before. But does that say more about you or that other person? If you knew someone had been the victim of a crime or abuse before, would that make you want to take advantage of them or help them?

> ▶▶ To watch a video to review what you just read here about trust, go to the CPT Whiteboard Video Library (*http://cptforptsd.com/cpt-resources*) and watch the video called *Trust II: Self and Others*.

 ## PRACTICE ASSIGNMENT

Look over your Stuck Point Log (page 56) to pick out the stuck points that are concerned with self- or other-trust. If you have issues with self- or other-trust, complete Alternative Thoughts Worksheets on them (see pages 199–205). Also notice whether you still have any stuck points about why the trauma happened related to trust—for example, "The trauma happened because I trusted that person" or "It happened because I had bad judgment." If so, do those first.

 ## TROUBLESHOOTING

I'm still stuck. I'm having a hard time letting go of my trust beliefs.

If you're having a hard time letting go of your trust beliefs like "If I trust someone, I will be hurt," consider whether you still have any related *trust beliefs about why your traumatic event occurred,* and if so, do those first. For example, if you're still thinking "The trauma happened because I trusted that person" or "If I had had better judgment, the trauma wouldn't have happened," then it would make sense that you are still thinking "I cannot trust anyone" or "I can't trust my judgment." However, reconsider the facts of the trauma. Did the trauma happen because you trusted someone, or did it happen because that person chose to hurt you? Did the trauma happen because you had bad judgment, or is there a better explanation for why it happened, like someone worked hard to deceive you and make you think they were trustworthy just so that they could hurt you? Go back and do an Alternative Thoughts Worksheet (pages 199–205) on the trust stuck point about why the trauma happened. Then see if you can make more progress on the more general stuck points about trust.

Is it worth it to ever trust anyone again?

How would things be different in your life if you let someone get close to you? What if they didn't end up betraying you? Would it have been worth it to trust them? It's likely that many good experiences can come from extending trust and building new relationships. But remember there are very few, if any, people we can trust in absolutely every way, so don't think of it as having to trust someone completely. Can they fly a plane, conduct eye surgery on you, bake you a good cake, or be good company? One of those may be all you need to trust, based on the kind of relationship you have. We trust different people with different things and extend different levels of trust. Important kinds of trust can take a long time to grow and, in fact, you may have people you already have in your life that you have been distrusting when you don't need to, and you just haven't given them a chance. There are people who don't need a lot of trust to engage in activities with. You don't have to entrust someone with your deepest secrets to go out to dinner or play a sport together. Learn about someone through your experiences with them and notice how they treat other people, strangers, friends, and family. Do other people like them and seem to trust them?

How do I know when to give people a second chance or when to let them go?

If someone makes a mistake like telling someone else something you told them, think back to whether you told them it was confidential. If you did and they betrayed your confidence, then you might talk to them about it and give them one more chance (with something smaller perhaps). If they betray your confidence again, you may not need to let them go from your life, but you won't want to tell them any more secrets. If you have experienced other kinds of trust violations, such as a romantic partner being unfaithful, being lied to repeatedly, or someone exploiting you financially, you may need to consider factors such as the context, the circumstances, the likelihood that it will continue to occur, and whether you want to try to allow them to rebuild trust. Those are very personal decisions that depend on many factors. The more experience you have with a person, the more you can move them up and down the line on the Trust Star (see page 187) depending on how they behave toward you.

The one exception is violence. You need to have a zero-tolerance policy with violence going forward. If someone is violent or verbally abusive with you or your family, one offense is enough to decide that they should no longer be a significant part of your life. Depending on the circumstances, you can cut off contact, or at least (in the case of people you may need to have some contact with, like your child's other parent) sharply limit contact with them. In these cases, getting help from a therapist or a domestic violence organization may be helpful in determining whether and how to have safe contact.

People tell me I need to forgive the person/people who harmed me, but I can't bring myself to.

Your beliefs on forgiveness are likely influenced by what your upbringing and perhaps your religion have told you. However, forgiveness is a highly personal decision. You are the one who can decide whether and when to forgive, and you can make this decision on your own timeline and after considering your own beliefs and values. One question to ask yourself is whether the person who offended you has even asked for forgiveness. Take some time to consider what forgiveness means to you, and how you came to believe what you do about forgiveness.

If the person who hurt you does not show remorse or try to change, they are not necessarily demonstrating that they are willing to do what it takes to rebuild trust or to have a relationship with you. Sometimes the harm that people have done is too substantial to make forgiveness seem possible. In such cases, acceptance may be a better goal to work toward. You can accept that it happened without forgiving and still move forward in your recovery.

You can also decide to forgive someone but not trust them in certain ways, or in any way, if the reality is that they haven't shown themselves to be trustworthy. You may feel more forgiving one day and then find yourself still feeling angry at them another day. That's natural, and it doesn't mean that you aren't making progress toward healing. Consider whether you have any stuck points around forgiveness that you need to work on, such as "If I don't forgive them, I'm a bad person" or "If I don't forgive them, I can't move forward with my life" or "If I forgive them, that means what they did was OK." Remember that you can also forgive without believing that what they did was OK; in fact, forgiveness wouldn't be necessary if they had not done something wrong! Consider doing an Alternative Thoughts Worksheet (pages 199–205) if you have any stuck points on forgiveness.

But if someone betrays you, shouldn't you keep your distance?

It depends and is ultimately up to you. Questions to consider are: Did you talk to them about the betrayal? Was the betrayal accidental or intentional? Did they show regret and never do it again? If they changed for you, or are working toward change, this could be someone you want in your life. It also depends on how serious the breach of trust was and what kind of relationship you want with that person. There are many kinds of relationships ranging from acquaintances to close friends to intimate partners. You may have different kinds of relationships with family members, and you can be closer or more distant with them depending on how they treat you and whether they change over time.

I can't get past the idea that if I hadn't trusted that person, it wouldn't have happened.

Go back to the questions in Chapter 7 (pages 79–89) about blaming yourself for the event. Have you done an Alternative Thoughts Worksheet on that stuck point yet? If not, do one now. It might also help to do one again even if you did one before. What does your trust of the person have to do with their harming you? Might they have harmed you anyway, even if you didn't trust them? Was the problem that you trusted them or that they betrayed your trust? Did you have a reason not to trust that person before the traumatic event happened? Who had the intent for what happened when the traumatic event occurred?

*   *   *

Continue to track your progress by filling out the PTSD Checklist and marking your score on your Graph for Tracking Your Weekly Scores on page 24. Remember that when your score gets below 20, you may want to assess whether you have worked on all of the stuck points you need to and are ready to move toward wrapping up. Whenever you're ready, you can go to the section called "Planning for the Conclusion of CPT" on page 264. Otherwise keep working on your stuck points. If you feel stuck, refer back to the section called "If You Are Not Noticing Change" in the "Reflecting on Your Progress" part of the book (pages 152–156) and reread earlier sections of the book as needed.

Alternative Thoughts Worksheet

A. Situation	B. Stuck point	D. Exploring thoughts	E. Thinking patterns	F. Alternative thought(s)
Describe the event leading to the stuck point or unpleasant emotion(s).	Write your stuck point related to the situation in Section A. Rate your belief in this stuck point from 0 to 100%. (How strongly do you believe this thought?)	Use the **exploring questions** to examine your automatic thought from Section B. Consider whether the thought is balanced and factual or extreme.	Use the **thinking patterns** to decide whether this is one of the patterns and explain why.	What else can you say instead of the thought in Section B? How else can you interpret the event instead of this thought? Rate your belief in the alternative thought(s) from 0 to 100%.
		Evidence against?	Jumping to conclusions:	
		What information is not included?	Ignoring important parts:	
		All or none? Extreme?	Oversimplifying/overgeneralizing:	
		Focused on just one piece of the event?		
		Questionable source of information?	Mind reading:	**G. Re-rate old stuck point** Re-rate how much you now believe the stuck point in Section B from 0 to 100%.
		Confusing possible with definite?		
	C. Emotion(s) Specify your emotion(s) (sad, angry, etc.) and rate how strongly you feel each emotion from 0 to 100%.	Based on feelings or facts?	Emotional reasoning:	**H. Emotion(s)** Now what do you feel? Rate from 0 to 100%.

Alternative Thoughts Worksheet

A. Situation	B. Stuck point		D. Exploring thoughts	E. Thinking patterns	F. Alternative thought(s)
Describe the event leading to the stuck point or unpleasant emotion(s).	Write your stuck point related to the situation in Section A. Rate your belief in this stuck point from 0 to 100%. (How strongly do you believe this thought?)		Use the **exploring questions** to examine your automatic thought from Section B. Consider whether the thought is balanced and factual or extreme.	Use the **thinking patterns** to decide whether this is one of the patterns and explain why.	What else can you say instead of the thought in Section B? How else can you interpret the event instead of this thought? Rate your belief in the alternative thought(s) from 0 to 100%.
			Evidence against?	Jumping to conclusions:	
			What information is not included?		
				Ignoring important parts:	
			All or none? Extreme?		
			Focused on just one piece of the event?	Oversimplifying/overgeneralizing:	
	C. Emotion(s) Specify your emotion(s) (sad, angry, etc.) and rate how strongly you feel each emotion from 0 to 100%.		Questionable source of information?	Mind reading:	**G. Re-rate old stuck point** Re-rate how much you now believe the stuck point in Section B from 0 to 100%.
			Confusing possible with definite?		
			Based on feelings or facts?	Emotional reasoning:	**H. Emotion(s)** Now what do you feel? Rate from 0 to 100%.

Alternative Thoughts Worksheet

A. Situation	B. Stuck point	D. Exploring thoughts	E. Thinking patterns	F. Alternative thought(s)
Describe the event leading to the stuck point or unpleasant emotion(s).	Write your stuck point related to the situation in Section A. Rate your belief in this stuck point from 0 to 100%. (How strongly do you believe this thought?)	Use the **exploring questions** to examine your automatic thought from Section B. Consider whether the thought is balanced and factual or extreme.	Use the **thinking patterns** to decide whether this is one of the patterns and explain why.	What else can you say instead of the thought in Section B? How else can you interpret the event instead of this thought? Rate your belief in the alternative thought(s) from 0 to 100%.
		Evidence against?	Jumping to conclusions:	
		What information is not included?	Ignoring important parts:	
		All or none? Extreme?		
		Focused on just one piece of the event?	Oversimplifying/overgeneralizing:	
C. Emotion(s) Specify your emotion(s) (sad, angry, etc.) and rate how strongly you feel each emotion from 0 to 100%.		Questionable source of information?	Mind reading:	**G. Re-rate old stuck point** Re-rate how much you now believe the stuck point in Section B from 0 to 100%.
		Confusing possible with definite?		
		Based on feelings or facts?	Emotional reasoning:	**H. Emotion(s)** Now what do you feel? Rate from 0 to 100%.

Alternative Thoughts Worksheet

A. Situation	B. Stuck point	C. Emotion(s)	D. Exploring thoughts	E. Thinking patterns	F. Alternative thought(s)
Describe the event leading to the stuck point or unpleasant emotion(s).	Write your stuck point related to the situation in Section A. Rate your belief in this stuck point from 0 to 100%. (How strongly do you believe this thought?)	Specify your emotion(s) (sad, angry, etc.) and rate how strongly you feel each emotion from 0 to 100%.	Use the **exploring questions** to examine your automatic thought from Section B. Consider whether the thought is balanced and factual or extreme.	Use the **thinking patterns** to decide whether this is one of the patterns and explain why.	What else can you say instead of the thought in Section B? How else can you interpret the event instead of this thought? Rate your belief in the alternative thought(s) from 0 to 100%.
			Evidence against?	Jumping to conclusions:	
			What information is not included?		
			All or none? Extreme?	Ignoring important parts:	
			Focused on just one piece of the event?	Oversimplifying/overgeneralizing:	
			Questionable source of information?	Mind reading:	**G. Re-rate old stuck point** Re-rate how much you now believe the stuck point in Section B from 0 to 100%.
			Confusing possible with definite?		
			Based on feelings or facts?	Emotional reasoning:	**H. Emotion(s)** Now what do you feel? Rate from 0 to 100%.

Alternative Thoughts Worksheet

A. Situation	B. Stuck point	C. Emotion(s)	D. Exploring thoughts	E. Thinking patterns	F. Alternative thought(s)	G. Re-rate old stuck point	H. Emotion(s)
Describe the event leading to the stuck point or unpleasant emotion(s).	Write your stuck point related to the situation in Section A. Rate your belief in this stuck point from 0 to 100%. (How strongly do you believe this thought?)	Specify your emotion(s) (sad, angry, etc.) and rate how strongly you feel each emotion from 0 to 100%.	Use the **exploring questions** to examine your automatic thought from Section B. Consider whether the thought is balanced and factual or extreme. Evidence against? What information is not included? All or none? Extreme? Focused on just one piece of the event? Questionable source of information? Confusing possible with definite? Based on feelings or facts?	Use the **thinking patterns** to decide whether this is one of the patterns and explain why. Jumping to conclusions: Ignoring important parts: Oversimplifying/overgeneralizing: Mind reading: Emotional reasoning:	What else can you say instead of the thought in Section B? How else can you interpret the event instead of this thought? Rate your belief in the alternative thought(s) from 0 to 100%.	Re-rate how much you now believe the stuck point in Section B from 0 to 100%.	Now what do you feel? Rate from 0 to 100%.

Alternative Thoughts Worksheet

A. Situation	B. Stuck point	C. Emotion(s)	D. Exploring thoughts	E. Thinking patterns	F. Alternative thought(s)	G. Re-rate old stuck point	H. Emotion(s)
Describe the event leading to the stuck point or unpleasant emotion(s).	Write your stuck point related to the situation in Section A. Rate your belief in this stuck point from 0 to 100%. (How strongly do you believe this thought?)	Specify your emotion(s) (sad, angry, etc.) and rate how strongly you feel each emotion from 0 to 100%.	Use the **exploring questions** to examine your automatic thought from Section B. Consider whether the thought is balanced and factual or extreme. Evidence against? What information is not included? All or none? Extreme? Focused on just one piece of the event? Questionable source of information? Confusing possible with definite? Based on feelings or facts?	Use the **thinking patterns** to decide whether this is one of the patterns and explain why. Jumping to conclusions: Ignoring important parts: Oversimplifying/overgeneralizing: Mind reading: Emotional reasoning:	What else can you say instead of the thought in Section B? How else can you interpret the event instead of this thought? Rate your belief in the alternative thought(s) from 0 to 100%.	Re-rate how much you now believe the stuck point in Section B from 0 to 100%.	Now what do you feel? Rate from 0 to 100%.

Alternative Thoughts Worksheet

A. Situation	B. Stuck point		D. Exploring thoughts	E. Thinking patterns	F. Alternative thought(s)
Describe the event leading to the stuck point or unpleasant emotion(s).	Write your stuck point related to the situation in Section A. Rate your belief in this stuck point from 0 to 100%. (How strongly do you believe this thought?)		Use the **exploring questions** to examine your automatic thought from Section B. Consider whether the thought is balanced and factual or extreme.	Use the **thinking patterns** to decide whether this is one of the patterns and explain why.	What else can you say instead of the thought in Section B? How else can you interpret the event instead of this thought? Rate your belief in the alternative thought(s) from 0 to 100%.
			Evidence against?	Jumping to conclusions:	
			What information is not included?	Ignoring important parts:	
			All or none? Extreme?		
			Focused on just one piece of the event?	Oversimplifying/overgeneralizing:	
			Questionable source of information?	Mind reading:	G. Re-rate old stuck point
			Confusing possible with definite?		Re-rate how much you now believe the stuck point in Section B from 0 to 100%.
	C. Emotion(s)			Emotional reasoning:	
	Specify your emotion(s) (sad, angry, etc.) and rate how strongly you feel each emotion from 0 to 100%.		Based on feelings or facts?		H. Emotion(s)
					Now what do you feel? Rate from 0 to 100%.

PTSD Checklist

Complete the PTSD Checklist to track your symptoms as you complete this book. Be sure to complete this measure on the same index event each time. When the instructions and questions refer to a "stressful experience," remember that that is your index event—the worst event that you are working on first.

Write in here the trauma that you are working on first: _____

Complete this PTSD Checklist with reference to that event.

Instructions: Below is a list of problems that people sometimes have in response to a very stressful experience. Please read each problem carefully, and then circle one of the numbers to the right to indicate how much you have been bothered by that problem *in the past week*.

In the past week, how much were you bothered by:	Not at all	A little bit	Mod- erately	Quite a bit	Extremely
1. Repeated, disturbing, and unwanted memories of the stressful experience?	0	1	2	3	4
2. Repeated, disturbing dreams of the stressful experience?	0	1	2	3	4
3. Suddenly feeling or acting as if the stressful experience were actually happening again (*as if you were actually back there reliving it*)?	0	1	2	3	4
4. Feeling very upset when something reminded you of the stressful experience?	0	1	2	3	4
5. Having strong physical reactions when something reminded you of the stressful experience (*for example, heart pounding, trouble breathing, sweating*)?	0	1	2	3	4
6. Avoiding memories, thoughts, or feelings related to the stressful experience?	0	1	2	3	4
7. Avoiding external reminders of the stressful experience (*for example, people, places, conversations, activities, objects, or situations*)?	0	1	2	3	4
8. Trouble remembering important parts of the stressful experience (not due to head injury or substances)?	0	1	2	3	4
9. Having strong negative beliefs about yourself, other people, or the world (*for example, having thoughts such as I am bad, There is something seriously wrong with me, No one can be trusted, or The world is completely dangerous*)?	0	1	2	3	4
10. Blaming yourself or someone else (who didn't intend the outcome) for the stressful experience or what happened after it?	0	1	2	3	4
11. Having strong negative feelings, such as fear, horror, anger, guilt, or shame?	0	1	2	3	4
12. Loss of interest in activities that you used to enjoy?	0	1	2	3	4
13. Feeling distant or cut off from other people?	0	1	2	3	4
14. Trouble experiencing positive feelings (*for example, being unable to feel happiness or have loving feelings for people close to you*)?	0	1	2	3	4
15. Irritable behavior, angry outbursts, or acting aggressively?	0	1	2	3	4
16. Taking too many risks or doing things that could cause you harm?	0	1	2	3	4
17. Being "super alert" or watchful or on guard?	0	1	2	3	4
18. Feeling jumpy or easily startled?	0	1	2	3	4
19. Having difficulty concentrating?	0	1	2	3	4
20. Trouble falling or staying asleep?	0	1	2	3	4

Add up the total and write it here: _____

13

Power and Control

Power and control are often a very big topic for people with PTSD. Traumatic events can challenge our beliefs about how much control we have over what happens to us. It can be a scary idea that traumatic events can happen in spite of our best efforts. Growing up in a society that perpetuates a just-world belief, you may have believed that you could generally control your own destiny by working hard and doing the "right" things. During the traumatic event, it's likely that you didn't have full (if any) control over what happened. This interacts with the just-world belief and can lead to stuck points about things you did or didn't do that you think caused or contributed to the trauma. By now, you have spent some time working on self-blame stuck points about the trauma, but if you still believe any of them, this is an important time to revisit them and do more Alternative Thoughts Worksheets on them (see pages 216–222).

Just as people develop stuck points around what they should have done differently at the time of the traumatic event, they may begin to form stuck points around what they need to do in the future to prevent bad things from happening again. After the traumatic event, you may have started to believe that you need to make sure you have complete control over what happens to you in the future. This may even extend to believing you need to try to control what other people in your life do, to help keep them or yourself safe. For example, some parents who struggle with PTSD may strictly limit their children's activities as a way of trying to keep them safe. All of these efforts to control can be quite exhausting and may be harmful to child development!

It makes sense that people want to feel in control if they didn't feel in control during the trauma. The problem is, while we have control over our own behaviors and actions in most situations, we can't control all of the factors that cause or contribute to traumas. We can't control whether there will be a natural disaster or whether someone else decides to commit a crime. We can't control other people's behaviors and reactions. We can't prevent every accident. It can be a scary idea that we can't prevent all traumatic events despite our best efforts.

Just as it would be going overboard to say, "I must be able to control every situation from now on," it's also going overboard to change your belief to "If I can't control everything around me, I have no control at all over what happens to me." The goal is to slow down and get a realistic understanding of what we can and can't control and what this means for us. Attempts at complete control don't succeed in the long run and will contribute to your PTSD, often in the form of other problems. With some perspective taking (and some Alternative Thoughts Worksheets), you can remember that most days are not filled with traumatic events—they are just ordinary days when nothing bad happens. It's easy to skip over the days in which nothing in particular happened as if they don't matter, but they count just as much. Other days, but not all days, are particularly positive or marked by our achieving some big goal. Count all days, not just the traumatic ones, to fill out the picture of your life.

As you do this work, you may notice power and control stuck points about yourself that are indirectly related to the trauma, such as "I have no control over what happens to me" (leading to feelings of fear and helplessness) or "I have to keep my emotions under control at all times" (leading to feelings of anger at yourself when you can't control your emotions or to avoidance of certain situations that might trigger difficult memories and emotions). You may have also formed power- and control-related stuck points about others, such as "There is no point in challenging people in positions of authority, even if they do something wrong" or "People will always try to exploit and control me" (leading to anger and helplessness).

Remember that power and control can also exist in multiple areas: You may have a lot of control over how neat your house is, when you go to bed, and what you eat, but less control over your work schedule or your partner's smoking habit. You can, however, control to some extent whether you decide to look for a different job and whether you spend time with your partner while they are smoking. Thinking about your relative power and control in different areas can help you feel less "all-or-none" about how much power and control you have, and it can also help you decide if there are areas where it might be good to give up some control or to take back some power.

Some people may have been living in circumstances that made them feel powerless even before the trauma. For example, children have much less power and control than adults, and, in abusive situations, there may be very little they can do. If this was true for you, later traumatic event(s) may have reinforced the belief that you have no control over what happens to you. This stuck point may lead you to be less assertive or to set and hold fewer boundaries with people in your life. When this happens, you can end up in situations that don't feel right for you and that can further reinforce your beliefs that you don't have control.

There are ways that people may give up power without even realizing that's what they're doing. For example, letting someone who is trying to manipulate you "push your buttons" means that you are letting them control your reactions. You can take back power by observing their behavior and taking a break without reacting, doing an Alternative Thoughts Worksheet (see pages 216–222) on stuck points that their behavior brings up for you, or working to remain calm and assertive as you respond to them. Another way that people sometimes give up power is by putting everyone else's needs before their own or not asking for help when they need it. While taking back power is very important for people who find themselves in these situations, it can take some practice to find the best ways to do this without taking power in less healthy ways.

Being assertive is a great example of a healthy way to take power, while being aggressive, testing people's limits, trying to manage their activities and behavior, and making unreasonable ultimatums are examples of unhealthy ways to develop a sense of power and control. Being assertive would involve stating your needs and wants clearly and respectfully, and saying "No" and setting limits when something doesn't feel right for you or fit with what you want to do. This requires being honest with yourself and others. For example, instead of putting your own needs and obligations aside, you could tell a friend who asks for a ride that you can't do it right now but you could do it if they could wait a couple of hours. Or it could mean telling your family that you don't feel like making dinner every night of the week and that you would like some help around the house.

Sometimes people are surprised or displeased when we set limits, but that doesn't mean it isn't the right thing for us to do. You don't need to justify or explain your limits to people who aren't respectful of them, and you don't need to change your boundaries because people don't like them. If you aren't sure if your limits are reasonable, try doing an Alternative Thoughts Worksheet on potential stuck points that come up for you like "I should be willing to change my plans to help them" or "If I set a limit, it means I'm selfish." Remember, too, that people sometimes appreciate when we are honest with them or give up some power by asking for their help. If you've been doing a lot for other people, it might make them feel good to be able to do some nice things for you in return.

Lack of control is often viewed as just a negative thing—however, you can give away power in positive ways. A small way to give up some control with low stakes might be telling your friend that they can choose the restaurant the next time you go out. They might appreciate it if you are usually the one deciding, and you have spared yourself the time it would take to look up different places to find out what they serve and whether they are open. It can also be very freeing to realize that you can control only your own actions, responses, and behaviors, and that you are not responsible for how others behave. This does not mean that you need to change your behavior if they react badly to your efforts to assert yourself. It just means that they have chosen to react badly, but you can remain firm about what you know is right for you. It can also be rewarding to share yourself, including your thoughts and feelings, with another person as part of the natural give-and-take in a healthy relationship. It can feel good to help others without expecting anything in return. These are examples of giving up some power in positive and healthy ways.

Another way to give up some power and control in a healthy way is to give up perfectionism. Sometimes you may take on too many responsibilities (cooking, cleaning up) because you think everything has to be done perfectly and other people in your life don't always do things the way you would. In these cases, you could give up some control and not try to have everything done "perfectly."

As you do worksheets on power and control, you may notice yourself getting better at doing them. You may also find that there are different ways to evaluate a single stuck point, such as rewording it or focusing on a different word in the stuck point. For example, perhaps you focused on the word *control* in the stuck point "If I don't have complete control over my spouse, something bad will happen to them." You may have considered different kinds of control and whether every kind is necessary for safety or focused on whether you need to have *complete* control. However, you could also examine the stuck point by focusing on the second half of the stuck point, that "something bad will happen to them," considering how this is jumping to conclusions and exaggerating the likelihood of harm. You can also develop multiple alternative thoughts that you can choose from that will lead to more balanced thinking and less intense emotions. In other words, you can do several worksheets on the same stuck point.

> Cynthia, who experienced multiple sexual assaults as an adolescent and adult after a history of sexual abuse as a child, had long believed that nobody would listen to her if she asserted herself. She found it very difficult to set boundaries with men that she dated, some of whom were verbally abusive or unfaithful. She felt unhappy, unsafe, and exploited in her relationships. Through her work using the skills and activities in CPT, she came to realize that power and control stuck points not only affected her relationships with men ("He won't take me seriously if I ask him to stop flirting with other women, so I just have to live with it") but also her work. She identified stuck points like "My coworkers and supervisors don't take me seriously" and "There is no point in rocking the boat" by saying, "No" when people asked her to take on duties that were not part of her job. As a result, she felt more and more demoralized. This made it difficult to ask her supervisor to assign some of her duties to others or ask for a raise or promotion.
>
> After Cynthia worked on her power and control stuck points related to the traumatic event itself, she began to work on stuck points in other areas of her life, like dating and work, and began to take back a sense of power and control. She became more assertive in her relationships, distancing herself from people who didn't respect the reasonable limits that she set. She worked on stuck points that came up as she took these important steps, and it helped her remain resolved when she doubted herself (which is often a habit for people who had experiences like Cynthia's). She also talked with her boss about changing her work duties and compensation and found that he was receptive to her requests and suggestions. She found that she felt stronger and more in control when she stated her limits, boundaries, and requests to others calmly and assertively. Even when people didn't respond the way she hoped, she recognized that she had choices about what she could do once she learned what their reactions were.

☑ Key Points on Power and Control

Just as safety and trust stuck points can occur with respect to ourselves and others and in multiple situations, so can beliefs about power and control. Consider ways that your past beliefs related to power and control may have shaped how you react to current situations.

Power and Control Related to Self

Power and control with respect to yourself is the belief that you can meet challenges that you may face and solve problems without being completely dependent on others.

⊃ If you grew up believing that you could handle problems and that you had control over what happened to you, the traumatic event may have disrupted that belief.

⊃ On the other hand, if you grew up in a situation where you didn't have much control, or where you experienced repeated and ongoing traumatic events, you may have developed the belief that the world is chaotic and uncontrollable, that you are helpless, and that many problems can't be solved through your own efforts.

As a result, you may feel numb, passive, hopeless, or depressed, and you might avoid situations and relationships that feel uncontrollable. You might also find yourself engaged in some self-destructive behaviors (for example, substance use, eating problems, spending sprees) that give you a temporary sense of control or a temporary feeling of having a break from stressful and uncontrollable situations. You might also find yourself experiencing rage, anger, or helplessness when people don't listen to you or behave in ways that you want them to.

Pretrauma belief	Posttrauma stuck points	Possible balanced/alternative thought
I have control over what happens to me.	I failed to control that situation, so I need to work even harder to keep everything in control.	While I'm not helpless or powerless, I can't always completely control other people or events.
I have control over myself.	I have to have complete control over my emotions and reactions.	Bad things do not always happen when I am not in complete control. While I'm not helpless or powerless, I can't always completely control my reactions (especially in extreme situations).
I have no control over what happens to me.	There's no point in trying to change what happens to me.	I can't control everything, especially other people, but I can control some aspects of what happens. I can decide to stay away from untrustworthy people. I can take precautions and set limits.
I am helpless.	I have no control over anything.	I make a lot of decisions in my everyday life, and many are good decisions. I can work on taking more control, being assertive, and doing what I think is right for me.

Power and Control Beliefs Related to Others

These beliefs center around the idea that you can control others or future events related to others, including people who have some form of power or authority. It also includes stuck points about the amount of power and control that people have over you.

⮑ If you had early experiences where you could influence the outcome of events, or if you had positive experiences with others, and you were not mistreated by others who were in some position of power or authority, you may have come to believe that it's possible to influence other people or events. The traumatic event(s) you experienced may have led you to believe, instead, that because you couldn't control the outcome of the event(s), you have no control or influence over people or events.

⮑ If you had previous experience with others that led you to believe that you were powerless in relation to others, or that other people will abuse power and authority and harm you, the traumatic event may have seemed to confirm those beliefs.

You may have come to believe that people will always try to control you or that there's no point in pushing back against people who abuse their power. As a result, you may find yourself being passive or submissive, not being assertive, or unable to maintain relationships because you don't allow others to exert any control in the relationship. Or instead, you might find yourself enraged when you see abuses of power.

Pretrauma belief	Posttrauma stuck points	Possible balanced/alternative thoughts
I have control over whether others mistreat me.	I need to stay on guard and in control with others so they don't harm or take advantage of me.	I can take steps to try to avoid being mistreated, but I can't control others' behavior or choices. I can choose to limit or end my contact with people who treat me badly if they aren't receptive to my feedback about it.
I have control over what happens in my relationships.	There is no point in trying to have control over how I am treated. I'm powerless.	Even though I cannot always get everything I want in a relationship or control how others treat me, I can influence others by standing up assertively for my rights and asking for what I want or need.
		A healthy relationship is one where people share and balance power. If it's not balanced, I can exert my control in this relationship by ending it if I need to. I can live with the disappointment and move on to find a healthier relationship when I'm ready.

Pretrauma belief	Posttrauma stuck points	Possible balanced/alternative thoughts
I don't have to worry about power or control imbalances in my relationships.	I have to control what happens in all of my relationships so I don't get hurt.	Even though I may not get everything I want or need out of a relationship, I can assert myself and ask for what I need. It can be OK to let others have some of the power in a relationship. It might even be helpful to have others take responsibility for some of the things that need to be done.
People in authority will [or won't] hurt me.	People in authority will always abuse their power and hurt or take advantage of me.	There are some people who will abuse their power. I also have examples of people who do not. If I see or experience abuses of power, I have some choices about what I do, including advocating, organizing, or fighting for change and having a plan for what to do if something happens to me (like if I am harmed, mistreated, or detained).

▶▶| To watch a video to review what you just read about power and control, go to the CPT Whiteboard Video Library (*http://cptforptsd.com/cpt-resources*) and watch the videos called *Power and Control Related to Self* and *Power and Control Related to Others.*

PRACTICE ASSIGNMENT

Look over your Stuck Point Log on page 56 to pick out the stuck points that are concerned with self- or other-power/control. If you have issues with self- or other-power/control, complete Alternative Thoughts Worksheets on them (see pages 216–222). Also notice whether you still have any stuck points about why the trauma happened related to power/control—for example, "I should have been more in control." If so, do those first.

TROUBLESHOOTING

I'm still stuck. I'm having a hard time letting go of my power/control beliefs.

If you're having a hard time letting go of your power/control beliefs like "If I'm not in total control, something terrible will happen," consider whether you still have any related *power/control beliefs about why your traumatic event occurred,* and if so, do those first. For example, if you're still thinking "I should have been more in control" or "It happened because I gave up my control," it would make sense that you are still thinking "I must always be in control." However, reconsider the facts of the trauma. Did the trauma happen because you gave up your control? Can anyone be in control one hundred percent of the time? Can bad things happen even when we think we are in control? Can people lack full control and still be safe? What actually has to be present to make a situation dangerous? Go back and do an Alternative Thoughts Worksheet on the power/control stuck point about why the trauma happened. Then see if you can make more progress on the general stuck points about power and control.

It can also be useful to ask yourself what it's costing you to try to remain in complete control. Is it limiting what you're doing in your everyday life? Does it affect your relationships with others? What would it mean to you to give up a small amount of control, in a situation where you are pretty sure (after doing some worksheets) that it would be safe to do so?

I have trouble asking people for help.

What's your stuck point about that? That they will refuse? That it will mean you are weak? That you will owe them? That someone will abuse you? The first step is to figure out why you have trouble asking people for help. What are your telling yourself? What outcomes are you expecting? Figure out your stuck points and then use an Alternative Thoughts Worksheet to explore them. If you can come up with an alternative thought you can believe, it'll become easier to ask people for help when you need it. Also consider what positive outcomes might result from asking for help.

It's so hard to let go of the urges to self-harm.

These kinds of urges are addictive because they work in the short term and may also be your go-to but harmful forms of coping. Some people self-harm in an effort to shut down emotions. If you remember from the beginning of this book, there is a feedback loop between the emotional part of the brain and the thinking part of the brain. By making yourself complete a worksheet when you have an urge to self-harm, you are activating the thinking part, which results in reduced functioning in the emotional part of your brain, resulting in experiencing emotions less strongly and thus less urge to self-harm. If you have an urge, grab a worksheet and don't do anything until you have completed a worksheet about whatever is bothering you. You can also look at stuck points like "I have no control over what I do when I have urges to harm myself."

I have trouble saying "No." If I assert myself, I'm afraid I'll be hurt.

Hurt by whom? By anyone in particular or everyone? Did you learn in childhood that you could not say "No" to adults? Is this a carryover core belief, or does it come from adult events? If you were the victim of repeated abuse, it makes sense that you may be afraid to assert yourself. But, if you are now safe and away from your abuser, you can examine this stuck point with a worksheet and then collect evidence by trying small ways of saying "No" (for example, about what TV show you want to watch or that you would prefer to go to a different restaurant for lunch with coworkers). Notice how harmless people react. Did they hurt you? Did they reject you?

You may need to do some worksheets on stuck points that come up for you when you are assertive. You can notice what happens when you calmly but firmly assert yourself ("I'm not comfortable doing that"). However, it's important to remember that if people react negatively to your boundaries, that doesn't mean you were wrong to set limits. It might mean that those are people who are unwilling to respect your boundaries, and that's information about how safe they are to trust or spend time with. You don't need to explain or justify yourself when you're assertive about your limits. You also don't need to back down and do things that aren't comfortable or fair for you to do for/with them. If others don't respect your limits, that's valuable information about whether they are healthy people to have in your life. If they are used to your giving in when they push you to do what they want, it may take some time and consistency in setting limits before they understand that you mean what you say, but stick with it and you'll notice changes in how people treat you over time!

How do I know what is the right amount of control to have?

There are many things you control every day, from whether to hit the snooze alarm to what to eat for breakfast, and so forth—hundreds or even thousands of choices that you have control of. You cannot control other people, however, any more than you can control the weather. There is no "right amount of control." But pay attention to the emotions you feel and how your levels of control are affecting your relationships. These may be clues to whether you are giving up too much control or trying to be too much in control.

What is the point of standing up for myself if I have no control over events?

Your stuck point is that you have no control over events. First, it may be helpful to reflect that you actually make thousands of decisions every day that you have control over. If you don't believe that, start to list your decisions tomorrow beginning with when you decide to get out of bed. If you are referring to having no control over future potential traumatic events, you may not control whether they occur, but you may have some control within the event. If your house caught on fire, you might be able to call the fire department, grab some valuables, or alert others. Those would all be indicators of having control within an out-of-control situation.

*   *   *

Complete another PTSD Checklist and continue to track your progress on your Graph for Tracking Your Weekly Scores on page 24. Remember that when your score gets below 20, you may want to assess whether you have worked on all of the stuck points you need to and are ready to move toward wrapping up. Whenever you're ready, you can go to the section called "Planning for the Conclusion of CPT" (see page 264). Otherwise keep working on your stuck points. If you feel stuck, refer back to the section called "If You Are Not Noticing Change" in the "Reflecting on Your Progress" part of the book (see pages 152–156) and reread earlier sections of the book as needed.

Alternative Thoughts Worksheet

A. Situation	B. Stuck point	C. Emotion(s)	D. Exploring thoughts	E. Thinking patterns	F. Alternative thought(s)
Describe the event leading to the stuck point or unpleasant emotion(s).	Write your stuck point related to the situation in Section A. Rate your belief in this stuck point from 0 to 100%. (How strongly do you believe this thought?)		Use the **exploring questions** to examine your automatic thought from Section B. Consider whether the thought is balanced and factual or extreme.	Use the **thinking patterns** to decide whether this is one of the patterns and explain why.	What else can you say instead of the thought in Section B? How else can you interpret the event instead of this thought? Rate your belief in the alternative thought(s) from 0 to 100%.
			Evidence against?	Jumping to conclusions:	
			What information is not included?	Ignoring important parts:	
			All or none? Extreme?		
			Focused on just one piece of the event?	Oversimplifying/overgeneralizing:	
		C. Emotion(s) Specify your emotion(s) (sad, angry, etc.) and rate how strongly you feel each emotion from 0 to 100%.	Questionable source of information?	Mind reading:	**G. Re-rate old stuck point** Re-rate how much you now believe the stuck point in Section B from 0 to 100%.
			Confusing possible with definite?		
			Based on feelings or facts?	Emotional reasoning:	**H. Emotion(s)** Now what do you feel? Rate from 0 to 100%.

Alternative Thoughts Worksheet

A. Situation	B. Stuck point	C. Emotion(s)	D. Exploring thoughts	E. Thinking patterns	F. Alternative thought(s)
Describe the event leading to the stuck point or unpleasant emotion(s).	Write your stuck point related to the situation in Section A. Rate your belief in this stuck point from 0 to 100%. (How strongly do you believe this thought?)		Use the **exploring questions** to examine your automatic thought from Section B. Consider whether the thought is balanced and factual or extreme.	Use the **thinking patterns** to decide whether this is one of the patterns and explain why.	What else can you say instead of the thought in Section B? How else can you interpret the event instead of this thought? Rate your belief in the alternative thought(s) from 0 to 100%.
			Evidence against?	Jumping to conclusions:	
			What information is not included?	Ignoring important parts:	
			All or none? Extreme?		
			Focused on just one piece of the event?	Oversimplifying/overgeneralizing:	
			Questionable source of information?	Mind reading:	**G. Re-rate old stuck point** Re-rate how much you now believe the stuck point in Section B from 0 to 100%.
		C. Emotion(s) Specify your emotion(s) (sad, angry, etc.) and rate how strongly you feel each emotion from 0 to 100%.	Confusing possible with definite?		
			Based on feelings or facts?	Emotional reasoning:	**H. Emotion(s)** Now what do you feel? Rate from 0 to 100%.

Alternative Thoughts Worksheet

A. Situation	B. Stuck point	D. Exploring thoughts	E. Thinking patterns	F. Alternative thought(s)
Describe the event leading to the stuck point or unpleasant emotion(s).	Write your stuck point related to the situation in Section A. Rate your belief in this stuck point from 0 to 100%. (How strongly do you believe this thought?)	Use the **exploring questions** to examine your automatic thought from Section B. Consider whether the thought is balanced and factual or extreme.	Use the **thinking patterns** to decide whether this is one of the patterns and explain why.	What else can you say instead of the thought in Section B? How else can you interpret the event instead of this thought? Rate your belief in the alternative thought(s) from 0 to 100%.
		Evidence against?	Jumping to conclusions:	
		What information is not included?	Ignoring important parts:	
		All or none? Extreme?		
		Focused on just one piece of the event?	Oversimplifying/overgeneralizing:	
	C. Emotion(s) Specify your emotion(s) (sad, angry, etc.) and rate how strongly you feel each emotion from 0 to 100%.	Questionable source of information?	Mind reading:	**G. Re-rate old stuck point** Re-rate how much you now believe the stuck point in Section B from 0 to 100%.
		Confusing possible with definite?		
		Based on feelings or facts?	Emotional reasoning:	**H. Emotion(s)** Now what do you feel? Rate from 0 to 100%.

Alternative Thoughts Worksheet

A. Situation	B. Stuck point	D. Exploring thoughts	E. Thinking patterns	F. Alternative thought(s)
Describe the event leading to the stuck point or unpleasant emotion(s).	Write your stuck point related to the situation in Section A. Rate your belief in this stuck point from 0 to 100%. (How strongly do you believe this thought?)	Use the **exploring questions** to examine your automatic thought from Section B. Consider whether the thought is balanced and factual or extreme.	Use the **thinking patterns** to decide whether this is one of the patterns and explain why.	What else can you say instead of the thought in Section B? How else can you interpret the event instead of this thought? Rate your belief in the alternative thought(s) from 0 to 100%.
		Evidence against?	Jumping to conclusions:	
		What information is not included?	Ignoring important parts:	
		All or none? Extreme?		
		Focused on just one piece of the event?	Oversimplifying/overgeneralizing:	
	C. Emotion(s) Specify your emotion(s) (sad, angry, etc.) and rate how strongly you feel each emotion from 0 to 100%.	Questionable source of information?	Mind reading:	**G. Re-rate old stuck point** Re-rate how much you now believe the stuck point in Section B from 0 to 100%.
		Confusing possible with definite?		
		Based on feelings or facts?	Emotional reasoning:	**H. Emotion(s)** Now what do you feel? Rate from 0 to 100%.

Alternative Thoughts Worksheet

A. Situation	B. Stuck point	D. Exploring thoughts	E. Thinking patterns	F. Alternative thought(s)
Describe the event leading to the stuck point or unpleasant emotion(s).	Write your stuck point related to the situation in Section A. Rate your belief in this stuck point from 0 to 100%. (How strongly do you believe this thought?)	Use the **exploring questions** to examine your automatic thought from Section B. Consider whether the thought is balanced and factual or extreme. Evidence against?	Use the **thinking patterns** to decide whether this is one of the patterns and explain why. Jumping to conclusions:	What else can you say instead of the thought in Section B? How else can you interpret the event instead of this thought? Rate your belief in the alternative thought(s) from 0 to 100%.
		What information is not included?	Ignoring important parts:	
		All or none? Extreme?		
	C. Emotion(s) Specify your emotion(s) (sad, angry, etc.) and rate how strongly you feel each emotion from 0 to 100%.	Focused on just one piece of the event?	Oversimplifying/overgeneralizing:	**G. Re-rate old stuck point** Re-rate how much you now believe the stuck point in Section B from 0 to 100%.
		Questionable source of information?	Mind reading:	
		Confusing possible with definite?		
		Based on feelings or facts?	Emotional reasoning:	**H. Emotion(s)** Now what do you feel? Rate from 0 to 100%.

Alternative Thoughts Worksheet

A. Situation	B. Stuck point		D. Exploring thoughts	E. Thinking patterns	F. Alternative thought(s)
Describe the event leading to the stuck point or unpleasant emotion(s).	Write your stuck point related to the situation in Section A. Rate your belief in this stuck point from 0 to 100%. (How strongly do you believe this thought?)		Use the **exploring questions** to examine your automatic thought from Section B. Consider whether the thought is balanced and factual or extreme.	Use the **thinking patterns** to decide whether this is one of the patterns and explain why.	What else can you say instead of the thought in Section B? How else can you interpret the event instead of this thought? Rate your belief in the alternative thought(s) from 0 to 100%.
			Evidence against?	Jumping to conclusions:	
			What information is not included?	Ignoring important parts:	
			All or none? Extreme?		
			Focused on just one piece of the event?	Oversimplifying/overgeneralizing:	
	C. Emotion(s) Specify your emotion(s) (sad, angry, etc.) and rate how strongly you feel each emotion from 0 to 100%.		Questionable source of information?	Mind reading:	**G. Re-rate old stuck point** Re-rate how much you now believe the stuck point in Section B from 0 to 100%.
			Confusing possible with definite?		
			Based on feelings or facts?	Emotional reasoning:	**H. Emotion(s)** Now what do you feel? Rate from 0 to 100%.

From Getting Unstuck from PTSD by Patricia A. Resick, Shannon Wiltsey Stirman, and Stefanie T. LoSavio. Copyright © 2023 The Guilford Press. Purchasers of this book can photocopy and/or download additional copies of this worksheet at www.guilford.com/resick2-forms for personal use or use with clients; see copyright page for details.

Alternative Thoughts Worksheet

A. Situation

Describe the event leading to the stuck point or unpleasant emotion(s).

B. Stuck point

Write your stuck point related to the situation in Section A. Rate your belief in this stuck point from 0 to 100%.

(How strongly do you believe this thought?)

C. Emotion(s)

Specify your emotion(s) (sad, angry, etc.) and rate how strongly you feel each emotion from 0 to 100%.

D. Exploring thoughts

Use the **exploring questions** to examine your automatic thought from Section B.

Consider whether the thought is balanced and factual or extreme.

Evidence against?

What information is not included?

All or none? Extreme?

Focused on just one piece of the event?

Questionable source of information?

Confusing possible with definite?

Based on feelings or facts?

E. Thinking patterns

Use the **thinking patterns** to decide whether this is one of the patterns and explain why.

Jumping to conclusions:

Ignoring important parts:

Oversimplifying/overgeneralizing:

Mind reading:

Emotional reasoning:

F. Alternative thought(s)

What else can you say instead of the thought in Section B? How else can you interpret the event instead of this thought? Rate your belief in the alternative thought(s) from 0 to 100%.

G. Re-rate old stuck point

Re-rate how much you now believe the stuck point in Section B from 0 to 100%.

H. Emotion(s)

Now what do you feel? Rate from 0 to 100%.

⟨ PTSD Checklist ⟩

Complete the PTSD Checklist to track your symptoms as you complete this book. Be sure to complete this measure on the same index event each time. When the instructions and questions refer to a "stressful experience," remember that that is your index event—the worst event that you are working on first.

Write in here the trauma that you are working on first: _____

Complete this PTSD Checklist with reference to that event.

Instructions: Below is a list of problems that people sometimes have in response to a very stressful experience. Please read each problem carefully, and then circle one of the numbers to the right to indicate how much you have been bothered by that problem *in the past week*.

In the past week, how much were you bothered by:	Not at all	A little bit	Mod-erately	Quite a bit	Extremely
1. Repeated, disturbing, and unwanted memories of the stressful experience?	0	1	2	3	4
2. Repeated, disturbing dreams of the stressful experience?	0	1	2	3	4
3. Suddenly feeling or acting as if the stressful experience were actually happening again (*as if you were actually back there reliving it*)?	0	1	2	3	4
4. Feeling very upset when something reminded you of the stressful experience?	0	1	2	3	4
5. Having strong physical reactions when something reminded you of the stressful experience (*for example, heart pounding, trouble breathing, sweating*)?	0	1	2	3	4
6. Avoiding memories, thoughts, or feelings related to the stressful experience?	0	1	2	3	4
7. Avoiding external reminders of the stressful experience (*for example, people, places, conversations, activities, objects, or situations*)?	0	1	2	3	4
8. Trouble remembering important parts of the stressful experience (not due to head injury or substances)?	0	1	2	3	4
9. Having strong negative beliefs about yourself, other people, or the world (*for example, having thoughts such as I am bad, There is something seriously wrong with me, No one can be trusted, or The world is completely dangerous*)?	0	1	2	3	4
10. Blaming yourself or someone else (who didn't intend the outcome) for the stressful experience or what happened after it?	0	1	2	3	4
11. Having strong negative feelings, such as fear, horror, anger, guilt, or shame?	0	1	2	3	4
12. Loss of interest in activities that you used to enjoy?	0	1	2	3	4
13. Feeling distant or cut off from other people?	0	1	2	3	4
14. Trouble experiencing positive feelings (*for example, being unable to feel happiness or have loving feelings for people close to you*)?	0	1	2	3	4
15. Irritable behavior, angry outbursts, or acting aggressively?	0	1	2	3	4
16. Taking too many risks or doing things that could cause you harm?	0	1	2	3	4
17. Being "super alert" or watchful or on guard?	0	1	2	3	4
18. Feeling jumpy or easily startled?	0	1	2	3	4
19. Having difficulty concentrating?	0	1	2	3	4
20. Trouble falling or staying asleep?	0	1	2	3	4

Add up the total and write it here: _____

From *PTSD Checklist for DSM-5 (PCL-5)* by Weathers, Litz, Keane, Palmieri, Marx, and Schnurr (2013). Available from the National Center for PTSD at *www.ptsd.va.gov*; in the public domain. Reprinted in *Getting Unstuck from PTSD* (Guilford Press, 2023). Purchasers of this book can photocopy and/or download additional copies of this worksheet at *www.guilford.com/resick2-forms* for personal use or use with clients; see copyright page for details.

14

Esteem

Trauma and PTSD can have a profound impact on people's sense of self-esteem and also on their esteem or regard for others. Just as with the other areas we've looked at, the traumatic event may have changed how you feel about yourself or others, or it may have reinforced the negative beliefs you already had. Either way, your sense of esteem can impact how you feel about yourself and others as you interact with the world.

~~~~~~~~~~~~~~~~~~~ Self-Esteem ~~~~~~~~~~~~~~~~~~~

Self-esteem is often an issue for people who have experienced traumatic events. PTSD and trauma can leave someone feeling worthless or broken. Some people who played a role in their trauma (for example, killing someone in combat or in self-defense) may judge themselves harshly and believe that they should not be around other people or that they don't deserve happiness. They may even have stuck points like "I'm a monster" or "I am a murderer." People who were sexually assaulted sometimes have stuck points like "I'm damaged" and "Nobody would want to be with me if they knew what happened to me." Sometimes people also assume that their traumatic event happened to them because of something negative about them—for example, being bad, stupid, weak, or unlovable.

Looking at your Stuck Point Log (page 56), what do you say about yourself as a result of the trauma? Do any of these stuck points apply to you?

❑ I'm worthless.

❑ I'm disgusting.

❑ I'm a terrible person.

❑ I'm broken.

❑ Nobody will want me.

❑ I'm incompetent.

❑ I'm a failure.

❑ I don't deserve to recover.

If you had good self-esteem before the traumatic event, it might have been undermined by the trauma, especially if you were treated badly by others after the trauma or if you blamed yourself. People may have engaged in victim blaming, telling you that you should have been more careful or done something to avoid or prevent what happened. This may have left you believing negative things about yourself. Sometimes people who experience sexual traumas think they are now "dirty" because of the trauma. They think about how they were violated and feel like they are still "tainted" by that person's touch. While disgust is a natural emotion for someone to feel if they have been sexually violated, it can be helpful to consider Are *you* disgusting because of what someone did to you? or Is your *perpetrator* disgusting because they did something wrong and disgusting to you? Sometimes it helps to consider that the body is constantly in flux, and new cells are dying and shedding all the time. If it has been more than a few months since your trauma, there is nowhere left on your body inside or out where the perpetrator touched you. Your cells have regenerated, and the old ones are gone.

If you already had low self-esteem even before the trauma, the trauma may have reinforced how you already thought about yourself. If you were physically or sexually abused, or were emotionally abused with cruel words and actions by family members, it's possible that their behavior and words ate away at your self-esteem and that the traumas that happened later seemed like more proof that you were not deserving of a happy life or feeling good about yourself. In fact, in the process of wondering why the traumatic event happened to you, you may have assumed its happening meant something about you. But it might tell us more about the perpetrator who intended the harm than it does about you. They are the one who sought out someone to harm. Other people would not, and did not do what they did, so what does it say about the perpetrator?

Adolescence is a time of great change and vulnerability, in which self-esteem is often challenged. Unfortunately, many traumatic events (rape, assaults, accidents, combat) occur during adolescence, which psychologically is not complete until about age twenty-four. So, at a time when someone is trying to figure out who they are and what they want to do with their lives, a traumatic event can pull the rug out from already shaky self-esteem and halt maturation.

Kiara had a history of physical and sexual abuse at the hands of her father and older brother. When her mother found out, she told Kiara that she must have been asking for it and that she should have been more modest and careful. In her work on the trauma, Kiara identified stuck points related to esteem, including "It happened because I was immodest" and "I am disgusting." She assigned all of the blame for the abuse to herself. She believed that because she wore only a T-shirt and underpants to bed, her father and brother felt tempted by her "immodesty." As she worked through her stuck points, she realized that many of her friends slept in similar clothing and were not molested by their family members. She did not view them as immodest or disgusting, and neither did anyone else she knew. If others wore the same things and remained safe, was it her clothing choices that had caused the abuse? Who had decided to do those things to her? What choices and decisions did her father and brother make? What did it say about them that they were willing to do such things to a young girl? Over time, Kiara's beliefs began to shift. She realized she was a typical kid who had done nothing wrong and that her father and brother were the people who had decided to harm her. Maybe it wasn't something about her at all, except that she happened to be the person who was there for them to target. She also decided that having something terrible happen to her that was beyond her control didn't make her disgusting. In fact, she began to realize all of the ways that she was resilient and strong for facing the trauma and continuing to try to move forward.

Remember, too, that the esteem you have for yourself and others isn't really one-dimensional. If you slow down and think about it, you might find some areas where you have more confidence in yourself, and others where you need to build esteem. You might be able to acknowledge that you are a talented cook, singer, student, or athlete, or that despite your trauma history you were able to do things you're proud of, while also recognizing that you could use some help with managing money or with comfortably talking with people you don't know well. Similarly, others you interact with are likely not all good or all bad—they are people with strengths and weaknesses. Working to have a balanced view of yourself and others can help you make better decisions about whether and in what ways to interact with people in your life, and it can also help you counter negative all-or-none thinking about yourself.

What are some things about yourself that you feel proud of or good about?

_____

_____

_____

_____

～～～ If Your Trauma Involved Intentionally ～～～ Harming Someone (Other Than in Self-Defense)

But what if you did intend harm to someone and now you have PTSD because of guilt or shame over your actions? Put the event back into context. Even if you did something that you now consider wrong, look back and consider the circumstances at the time. This exercise is not intended to excuse you out of hand—guilt may well be the appropriate emotion if you harmed someone with intention—but to help you understand your actions in the context in which they occurred. We call this *right-sizing*: some guilt or self-blame is appropriate when you intend to hurt someone, but you need to give yourself the chance to understand why, as well as how you have changed or matured after not being in that same situation anymore.

REFLECTION

If you intended harm, take the time to ask yourself the following questions and really reflect and write down the answers:

How old were you? People's brains, and particularly the reasoning part, don't finish developing until they are in their mid-twenties. Were you younger than that? Were you more impulsive then?

_____

_____

_____

_____

Under what conditions did the event take place? Were you around people who were also doing those things, so it seemed normal or acceptable to do them? Did you have good role models and support? Had you been a victim of similar things in the past? Were you under the influence of any substances? Were you coerced in any way?

_____

_____

_____

_____

Did you keep doing it? When and why did you stop? Would you make the same decisions now?

_____

_____

_____

_____

Consider all of the other days in your life: the good days, the neutral days, and the bad days. Yes, some days are more important than others, but they all count as part of someone's life. Are you the same person with the same values as you were at the time of the event? Did you make a decision to do things differently at some point?

_____

_____

_____

_____

If you say things to yourself like "I'm a monster because I did that" or "I'm a terrible person because I was capable of doing that," ask yourself, "Do monsters feel remorse? Do people who do terrible things ever decide to change?"

_____

_____

_____

_____

One of the alternative thoughts to consider is "This event doesn't mean I am a bad person" or "I did something that I regret, but I have not continued to do things like that my whole life." Some people decide to do something to make amends to those they have harmed as part of their commitment to change. Others may have experienced legal consequences. If you have, how much longer and in what other ways is it really necessary to continue to pay for what you did? Are you giving yourself a life sentence? An important thing to consider is who you are now and who you want to be. It's important to look at your accomplishments, your kindnesses and the good things you've done, all the days when you weren't doing things you regret, and your efforts to change as part of a greater whole that is your life. One incident, or even a period of your life, does not completely define who you are now. An alternative thought might be "Good people can do bad things" or "People can change, and I have made different choices since I did that thing I regret."

~~~~~~~~~~~~~~~~~~ Esteem for Others ~~~~~~~~~~~~~~~~~~

Esteem for others has to do with your regard and beliefs about other people, often entire groups of people. Saying that "all men are bad" after being raped by a man is an example of an other-esteem stuck point. The statement "All people from that country are trying to kill us" by someone whose friend was killed while serving in the military during a war is another example of an other-esteem stuck point. In both cases, these are overgeneralizations from one person or situation to everyone in that group. One exception will prove that the statement is incorrect and will show that we need to think about people as individuals. Just as you can't decide right away whether or not you can trust someone you've just met, you can't decide whether to hold someone in high or low esteem until you've gotten to know more about them as individuals.

Maria, who you read about in Chapter 12 on trust, understandably had negative beliefs about people in authority after seeing that authority figures didn't always step in and help when she or her family were being harassed or attacked. When she moved to a different area than where she grew up, she noticed people had a broader range of attitudes. She saw that some of her bosses were welcoming and appreciated what she contributed and that they posted signs supporting immigrants in their windows during a time of political controversy around immigration-related issues. Even though she knew not "everyone" in authority abused their power, she understandably still felt anxious about what could happen to her, and she was having flashes of her brother's assault pop into her head each day and had difficulty sleeping. As Maria worked through her trauma, she gave fault and blame to the perpetrators of her brother's assault, as well as responsibility to other individuals who were in positions of authority who did not intervene quickly to help. What happened, and how some others responded, was not acceptable. She let herself feel the sadness about the event and anger at those who were involved or didn't step in to help. As she processed the event, the intrusive memories popped up less often and she was able to focus on the people and activities around her. Even though she didn't blindly trust authority figures or assume they would have her back, she was working on building new relationships in her life outside of her family, such as with her new boss and with a teacher from an expressive writing course she was taking who encouraged her to write about her story. She also developed a safety plan for what she would do if she or someone she cared about was in danger.

Building Esteem

In this chapter, in addition to completing worksheets on your esteem-related stuck points, you'll see two activities to help you build esteem and gather information to help you examine and change your stuck points. You'll learn about them after the Key Points on the Topic of Esteem, but feel free to read ahead to the Practice Assignment and start doing them as soon as possible. Hopefully, you'll find them to be a little different and a nice addition to your days.

☑ Key Points on the Topic of Esteem

Trauma can change one's esteem for themselves, or for others, or it can reinforce beliefs that were formed earlier in life. Consider how the points below relate to your own sense of esteem.

Esteem Beliefs Related to Self

Self-esteem is the belief in your own worth. All humans need to have a sense of self and self-worth. We develop self-esteem when we feel understood, respected, and taken seriously by the people in our lives.

➲ If your earlier experiences were positive and contributed to beliefs of self-worth, the traumatic event may disrupt those beliefs and lower your self-esteem. Your confidence in your ability to make good decisions for yourself and your confidence in your ideas and opinions may also suffer.

➲ If you had previous experiences that led to self-doubt and a poor sense of self-worth, traumatic events may have confirmed these negative beliefs about yourself.

Examples of life experiences that may have led to negative beliefs about yourself include hearing and believing negative things that other people said to and about you, not having much care or support from important people in your life, or being criticized and blamed for things that were not your fault.

These experiences can lead to beliefs such as "I am bad/evil," "I am damaged," "I am worthless," or "I deserve to have bad things happen to me." These stuck points can contribute to feelings of depression, shame, and guilt, and may also lead to harmful or self-destructive behavior.

Pretrauma belief	Posttrauma stuck points	Possible balanced/alternative thoughts
Bad things won't happen to me because I am a good person.	I did something to deserve it.	Anyone can have bad things happen to them. What happened may not have anything to do with whether I was good or bad.
I am fundamentally a worthy person.	I am damaged. Nobody will want to be with me.	Things that happen to me have an effect on me, but they don't define me. Many people experience trauma, and it doesn't mean that they are flawed or damaged. It means they are survivors.
I'm worthless.	I don't deserve to be treated well.	Even though I cannot always get everything I want in a relationship or control how others treat me, I can influence others by standing up assertively for my rights and asking for what I want or need.
I am worthy and deserving.	I don't deserve to have good things happen.	I didn't do anything that would make me unworthy of love. Even if I did some things I regret at times, it doesn't make me fundamentally undeserving.

Esteem Beliefs Related to Others

Other-related esteem beliefs focus on how much you value, or the regard you have for other people. Having a realistic view of people is important for how you interact with them and how you behave in relationships.

➲ If your previous experiences taught you that people are generally good and caring, experiences like the trauma or people's reactions to the trauma (such as their being blaming and unsupportive) may have undermined that belief in a significant way.

⮑ If you had previous experiences in which people exploited you, betrayed your trust, or harmed you, the trauma may have confirmed beliefs that people are fundamentally untrustworthy or harmful. If people in positions of authority were the ones who harmed you or contributed to harm, or if people from a specific background, gender, race, or ethnicity harmed you, you may begin to believe that everyone like that wants to exploit or harm you.

It's important to try to use all of the information available to you to examine these beliefs and assumptions. Beliefs that are rigid, stereotyped, or can't be changed even with new information limit the type and quality of relationships and can lead to cynicism, suspicion, bitterness, conflict, withdrawal, and isolation. Part of recovery is considering the costs of holding on to old patterns and beliefs and deciding what you want for yourself moving forward. What are the costs of holding on to these beliefs?

Pretrauma belief	Posttrauma stuck points	Possible balanced/alternative thoughts
People are generally good.	People don't care and are only out for themselves.	People are all different. Some are kind and caring most of the time, and others aren't. If I act as though everyone doesn't care, I might miss out on having healthy friendships and relationships.
People in authority will [or won't] hurt me.	People in authority will abuse their power and hurt or take advantage of me.	There are some people who will abuse their power and cause unfair things to happen. I also have examples of people who do not abuse power. It can make sense to be cautious based on my past experience, but I can observe how people in authority act to see what their intentions are.
People of that gender/race/ethnicity/political party are bad.	They are out to harm me.	Even though it makes sense to be cautious in light of my past experiences, I need to look at the full context for each individual person and situation rather than make a generalization about *everyone* with those characteristics.

▶▶ To watch a video to review what you just read here about esteem, go to the CPT Whiteboard Video Library (*http://cptforptsd.com/cpt-resources*) and watch the videos called *Self-Esteem* and *Other-Esteem*.

PRACTICE ASSIGNMENT, PART 1:
ALTERNATIVE THOUGHTS WORKSHEETS

Look over your Stuck Point Log on page 56 to pick out the stuck points that are concerned with self- or other-esteem to complete worksheets on. If you have issues with self- or other-esteem, complete Alternative Thoughts Worksheets on them (see pages 240–246). Also notice whether you still have any stuck points about why the trauma happened related to esteem—for example, "The trauma happened because I was weak." If so, do those first.

PRACTICE ASSIGNMENT, PART 2:
DOING SOMETHING NICE FOR YOURSELF EACH DAY

Also, begin doing one nice thing for yourself every day. It doesn't have to be something big or expensive—just take some time to do something you enjoy or that makes you feel good. Some people start spending more time with friends, doing an activity they used to enjoy but have stopped doing, or treating themselves to a food they like.

What if you don't have much time because you have work, school, or caregiving responsibilities? The goal can be to just carve out a few minutes for yourself. Some people decide to take fifteen minutes or so to read a book or magazine or take a walk before they get in their car to return home from work to relieve their babysitter. Others decide to let their kids watch a show or play independently for twenty or thirty minutes while they take some time to relax. Some people work with their network of friends and family to arrange for an hour or two to take a break. Whatever you do, you should make sure that the nice thing you do for yourself isn't something you have to "earn" by doing enough work or chores or other obligations. This is something you do for yourself with no conditions. Try having a plan for each day, with a backup activity or plan in case the first one doesn't work for some reason. Put a reminder on your phone or calendar if you need to or ask a supportive person in your life to help you remember and hold you accountable.

On the Log of Nice Things I Did for Myself on the facing page, write down some nice things you'll do for yourself and when. Then come back and check off whether you did them. If you notice stuck points like "I don't deserve this" or "I'm wasting time/money on myself"—you guessed it!—do a worksheet on those stuck points. You can also download and print the Log of Nice Things I Did for Myself from *www.guilford.com/resick2-forms*.

PRACTICE ASSIGNMENT, PART 3:
GIVING AND RECEIVING COMPLIMENTS

Additionally, each day, practice giving and receiving compliments, and use the Log of Compliments Given and Received on page 235 to keep track of them. You can also download and print the Log of Compliments Given and Received from *www.guilford.com/resick2-forms*. Why are we asking you to do this? People with PTSD often isolate. This means that they

Log of Nice Things I Did for Myself

Activity	Date	Completed?	Stuck points?

don't see as many people and may not be aware of people's reactions to them. If you have been very isolated, or if your relationships have suffered because of your PTSD, it may take some time to begin to notice or receive compliments. You may need to get out into the world more, make it a point to speak with other people, and do things that make you feel good about how you are treating people. When receiving compliments, it's important not to filter out or minimize nice things people say to you. They may be more objective about you than you are, and if you reject the compliment, they may be less likely to say nice things to you in the future, either because they don't want to make you feel uncomfortable or because they feel surprised or hurt that you rejected a compliment. If you notice any stuck points about the compliments you receive ("They don't mean it"), add them to your Stuck Points Log and use Alternative Thoughts Worksheets to evaluate them. A number of blank Alternative Thoughts Worksheets are provided on pages 240–246. And practice just saying, "Thank you" instead of minimizing the compliments! Try to incorporate what nice things other people say about you into your self-concept.

Giving compliments may help you with other-esteem. You might notice new evidence that people are doing good or kind things. For people you don't know well, try to focus your compliments on what they do or are good at, rather than complimenting aspects of appearance, which can make some people uncomfortable in some circumstances. Notice what other people are doing, and don't filter out what group they are from and whether they are doing something that is deserving of a compliment. Too often people do nice things that go unnoticed, and it's an opportunity for you to look around and see when people do something well or kind and to acknowledge it. It's a safe way to interact with people, and it's a good way to start expanding your interactions with other people.

You can use the Alternative Thoughts Worksheets to examine any stuck points that come up related to doing nice things for yourself, giving or receiving compliments, or other esteem-related stuck points. Be sure to also use them on any stuck points that are on your Stuck Point Log that you haven't resolved, especially if they focus on why the trauma happened.

 TROUBLESHOOTING

I'm still stuck. I'm having a hard time letting go of my esteem beliefs.

If you're having a hard time letting go of your esteem beliefs like "I'm weak" or "I'm unlovable," consider whether you still have any related *esteem beliefs about why your traumatic event occurred,* and if so, do those first. For example, if you're still thinking "The trauma happened because I was unlovable" or "If I had been stronger, the trauma wouldn't have happened," it would make sense that you are still thinking "I'm unlovable" and "I'm weak." However, reconsider the facts of the trauma. Did the trauma happen because you were unlovable, or did it happen because that person chose to hurt you? Does the fact that the trauma happened say more about you or the perpetrator, if there was one? If there wasn't a perpetrator, did it say more about you or the circumstances? Did the trauma happen because you were weak or stupid, or is there a better explanation for why it happened, such as someone choosing to do

Log of Compliments Given and Received

Date	Compliment	Given or received?	Stuck points

it? Go back and do a worksheet on the esteem stuck point about why the trauma happened. Then see if you can make more progress on the more general stuck points about esteem.

My self-esteem isn't changing after doing the worksheets.

Be patient with yourself. You've formed habits of thinking about yourself, which may be deeply rooted core beliefs, and it can take a while to undo them. The first step is to recognize those stuck points and do the exercises regularly. Pay more attention to what your friends and the people you trust and respect say than what you have been telling yourself for so long. Self-esteem stuck points are likely to be core beliefs, so they will have to be evaluated with regard not only to the traumatic events but also to everyday events. You may have a filter up like a set of blinds in a window that allows you to take in only information that matches your negative core belief about yourself. Everything that doesn't fit with your core beliefs either bounces off or is twisted around to fit your stuck point. You'll need to open up the blinds and allow all of the information in, not just the filtered thoughts that match your old beliefs.

I don't believe people when they compliment me. They don't know the real me.

That's a stuck point. Do you have it on your log? It's possible that they know more about the real you than you realize because they have seen how you treat people and how you act around them. Perhaps you have been in the habit of thinking you are worthless or blameworthy. People outside of you who can see your behavior may have a very different opinion based on their experiences with you. The "real" you is how you treat others and yourself today.

People don't like my compliments.

If someone reacted negatively to your compliment, consider the type of compliment. Was it on their appearance or on something they did? Some people are uncomfortable with compliments about their appearance, but they may appreciate having their hard work or kindness acknowledged. Or, is it possible that they have self-esteem issues that may make it difficult to accept the compliment? Try again with others and make sure you take all of their reactions into account as you continue with this exercise. People might not always react the way we hope, but there are many reasons that they might not react positively. Notice how different people react rather than focusing only on times that it doesn't go well. Also pay attention to any stuck points that come up for you. Are you jumping to conclusions about what their reactions mean? Are there other explanations for how they reacted, such as their own state of mind, stuck points, or thinking patterns?

I am so damaged that it's permanent.

This is a common stuck point. Hopefully by this point you are starting to question that kind of thinking. Ask yourself whether you really believe that other people who experienced terrible things through no fault of their own are damaged or irredeemable. If it happened to a friend, would you think of your friend that way? Did their trauma define who they are? Do you truly believe that people have to be free of trauma or hardship to be worthy of love and respect? Are there ways in which people who experienced traumatic events use resilience to get by in their everyday life? What are other things about you besides your trauma? Would people say things about your kindness, your work ethic, and your abilities? You can also ask yourself whether the fallout from the trauma is permanent and unchangeable. If you've noticed changes in your PTSD symptoms, stuck points, or mood, you already can see that nothing needs to be permanent. Remember that you got stuck in your PTSD, and when you get unstuck, you'll be on the road to recovery.

I don't deserve to do nice things for myself.

This stuck point usually follows self-blame or grief. Is there a part of one of your traumatic events for which you still blame yourself and have judged yourself so harshly that you think you don't deserve a good life? Is saying this a habit you developed because other people said or implied that you didn't deserve anything good? Consider the source and what their reasons might have been for saying those things.

One special case of this is when someone dies in the traumatic event. If someone you cared about died, then you may have decided that it would be disloyal to enjoy your life or do nice things for yourself because they can't. This idea can persist even if you've let go of the blame and hindsight bias that you should have been able to save that person. What would they want for you? If the situation were reversed, what would you want for them—to be miserable forever or to go on and have a good life? Is having PTSD the best way to honor someone? What about the alternative way to honor their life by living a good life for both of you? Which of these would you want for loved ones that you leave behind?

Another special case is having PTSD from perpetrating a crime or a traumatic event. If you need to, go back to examining your role in the event in Chapter 7 (pages 81–83). It may be possible that you are still taking on unnecessary blame. But if you did have intent, then you need to decide what to do with your guilt. You may be giving yourself a life sentence that may go way beyond what a judge would give (or did give). Are you the same person now that you were then? Did you have a choice then? What was the context? The very fact that you have had PTSD is proof that you are not a "monster"—would a monster experience regret or remorse? At this point you may want to focus on not just doing nice things for yourself but doing good things for others. Consider being a good citizen and giving back to your community. Volunteer work, for example, at an animal shelter, hospital, or homeless shelter, is giving back or taking positive action, especially if making amends directly isn't possible.

I know that not everyone is bad, but I don't want to take the risk.

You probably explored similar stuck points in Chapters 11 and 12, on safety and trust, respectively, and maybe again in Chapter 13 on power and control. If you are still facing this stuck point with other-esteem, the question is why you've condemned an entire group or population for the actions of one or a few. What is that core belief—that all people from a particular group are bad—costing you? Are you ignoring the exceptions and not even giving people the chance to show that it isn't the whole group or population that committed the traumatic event? Maybe the group is not even relevant to why the event happened. Are you overgeneralizing about members of a group to achieve that impossible goal of prediction and control? Hopefully by now if your PTSD symptoms have decreased, you can see that if some other negative event happens in your life, you can overcome it. Avoiding all people to potentially avoid one bad person means that you lose many wonderful people who could enrich your life. As in Chapter 11, this is a matter of probabilities and whether you want to sacrifice the many for one possible bad outcome.

I have been thinking this way for so long about that group of people that it is hard to think differently.

That is understandable. If you say something long enough it sounds like *truth,* and it becomes a habit to think that way. However, it's just an automatic thought, and if you look at it closely and frequently, you may start to change your mind. It's a process that may take many Alternative Thoughts Worksheets in many different situations. You most likely have been looking only for the evidence or the news on TV and media that fits your old viewpoint and disregarding all the other evidence against your thought. You may need to begin to try to understand more about people who are different from you: their experiences, beliefs, hopes, and communities. It may take a lot of practice to change your mind, but learning to think flexibly instead of rigidly will make the rest of your life much less anger filled, guilt ridden, or fear based, so you can turn to growth instead of running in place.

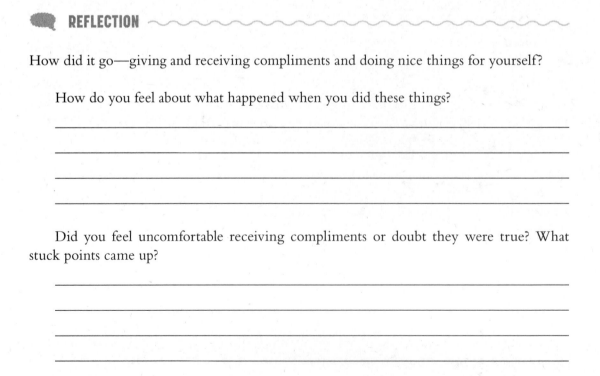 **REFLECTION**

How did it go—giving and receiving compliments and doing nice things for yourself?

How do you feel about what happened when you did these things?

_____

_____

_____

_____

Did you feel uncomfortable receiving compliments or doubt they were true? What stuck points came up?

_____

_____

_____

_____

Did you feel uncomfortable doing nice things for yourself? Why or why not?

_____

_____

_____

_____

Did you notice new or old stuck points coming up as you did these things? Which ones?

_____

_____

_____

_____

If so, did you do an Alternative Thoughts Worksheet on them?

_____

What did you learn from these activities?

_____

_____

_____

_____

These are assignments for life. It's a good idea to practice listening to compliments you receive with an open mind and notice when other people deserve a compliment. You should also make it a practice to have some time for yourself every day to do something you enjoy or find worthwhile. You may have forgotten what activities you like and how you would like to spend your free time. Try some new activities that you wouldn't try due to PTSD and keep working with any stuck points that come up along the way.

*   *   *

Complete another PTSD Checklist and continue to track your progress by filling out the Graph for Tracking Your Weekly Scores on page 24. Remember that when your score gets below 20 you may want to assess whether you have worked on all of the stuck points you need to and are ready to move toward wrapping up CPT. Whenever you're ready, you can go to the section called "Planning for the Conclusion of CPT" (page 264). Otherwise keep working on your stuck points. If you feel stuck, refer back to the section called "If You Are Not Noticing Change" in the "Reflecting on Your Progress" part of the book (pages 152–156) and reread earlier sections of the book as needed.

Alternative Thoughts Worksheet

A. Situation	B. Stuck point	C. Emotion(s)	D. Exploring thoughts	E. Thinking patterns	F. Alternative thought(s)
Describe the event leading to the stuck point or unpleasant emotion(s).	Write your stuck point related to the situation in Section A. Rate your belief in this stuck point from 0 to 100%. (How strongly do you believe this thought?)	Specify your emotion(s) (sad, angry, etc.) and rate how strongly you feel each emotion from 0 to 100%.	Use the **exploring questions** to examine your automatic thought from Section B. Consider whether the thought is balanced and factual or extreme. Evidence against? What information is not included? All or none? Extreme? Focused on just one piece of the event? Questionable source of information? Confusing possible with definite? Based on feelings or facts?	Use the **thinking patterns** to decide whether this is one of the patterns and explain why. Jumping to conclusions: Ignoring important parts: Oversimplifying/overgeneralizing: Mind reading: Emotional reasoning:	What else can you say instead of the thought in Section B? How else can you interpret the event instead of this thought? Rate your belief in the alternative thought(s) from 0 to 100%. **G. Re-rate old stuck point** Re-rate how much you now believe the stuck point in Section B from 0 to 100%. **H. Emotion(s)** Now what do you feel? Rate from 0 to 100%.

Alternative Thoughts Worksheet

A. Situation	B. Stuck point	C. Emotion(s)	D. Exploring thoughts	E. Thinking patterns	F. Alternative thought(s)
Describe the event leading to the stuck point or unpleasant emotion(s).	Write your stuck point related to the situation in Section A. Rate your belief in this stuck point from 0 to 100%. (How strongly do you believe this thought?)		Use the **exploring questions** to examine your automatic thought from Section B. Consider whether the thought is balanced and factual or extreme.	Use the **thinking patterns** to decide whether this is one of the patterns and explain why.	What else can you say instead of the thought in Section B? How else can you interpret the event instead of this thought? Rate your belief in the alternative thought(s) from 0 to 100%.
			Evidence against?	Jumping to conclusions:	
			What information is not included?	Ignoring important parts:	
			All or none? Extreme?		
			Focused on just one piece of the event?	Oversimplifying/overgeneralizing:	
		C. Emotion(s) Specify your emotion(s) (sad, angry, etc.) and rate how strongly you feel each emotion from 0 to 100%.	Questionable source of information?	Mind reading:	**G. Re-rate old stuck point** Re-rate how much you now believe the stuck point in Section B from 0 to 100%.
			Confusing possible with definite?		
			Based on feelings or facts?	Emotional reasoning:	**H. Emotion(s)** Now what do you feel? Rate from 0 to 100%.

Alternative Thoughts Worksheet

A. Situation	B. Stuck point	C. Emotion(s)	D. Exploring thoughts	E. Thinking patterns	F. Alternative thought(s)
Describe the event leading to the stuck point or unpleasant emotion(s).	Write your stuck point related to the situation in Section A. Rate your belief in this stuck point from 0 to 100%. (How strongly do you believe this thought?)	Specify your emotion(s) (sad, angry, etc.) and rate how strongly you feel each emotion from 0 to 100%.	Use the **exploring questions** to examine your automatic thought from Section B. Consider whether the thought is balanced and factual or extreme.	Use the **thinking patterns** to decide whether this is one of the patterns and explain why.	What else can you say instead of the thought in Section B? How else can you interpret the event instead of this thought? Rate your belief in the alternative thought(s) from 0 to 100%.
			Evidence against?	Jumping to conclusions:	
			What information is not included?	Ignoring important parts:	
			All or none? Extreme?	Oversimplifying/overgeneralizing:	
			Focused on just one piece of the event?		
			Questionable source of information?	Mind reading:	**G. Re-rate old stuck point** Re-rate how much you now believe the stuck point in Section B from 0 to 100%.
			Confusing possible with definite?		
			Based on feelings or facts?	Emotional reasoning:	**H. Emotion(s)** Now what do you feel? Rate from 0 to 100%.

Alternative Thoughts Worksheet

A. Situation	B. Stuck point	C. Emotion(s)	D. Exploring thoughts	E. Thinking patterns	F. Alternative thought(s)	G. Re-rate old stuck point	H. Emotion(s)
Describe the event leading to the stuck point or unpleasant emotion(s).	Write your stuck point related to the situation in Section A. Rate your belief in this stuck point from 0 to 100%. (How strongly do you believe this thought?)	Specify your emotion(s) (sad, angry, etc.) and rate how strongly you feel each emotion from 0 to 100%.	Use the **exploring questions** to examine your automatic thought from Section B. Consider whether the thought is balanced and factual or extreme.	Use the **thinking patterns** to decide whether this is one of the patterns and explain why.	What else can you say instead of the thought in Section B? How else can you interpret the event instead of this thought? Rate your belief in the alternative thought(s) from 0 to 100%.	Re-rate how much you now believe the stuck point in Section B from 0 to 100%.	Now what do you feel? Rate from 0 to 100%.
			Evidence against?	Jumping to conclusions:			
			What information is not included?	Ignoring important parts:			
			All or none? Extreme?				
			Focused on just one piece of the event?	Oversimplifying/overgeneralizing:			
			Questionable source of information?	Mind reading:			
			Confusing possible with definite?				
			Based on feelings or facts?	Emotional reasoning:			

Alternative Thoughts Worksheet

A. Situation	B. Stuck point	C. Emotion(s)	D. Exploring thoughts	E. Thinking patterns	F. Alternative thought(s)
Describe the event leading to the stuck point or unpleasant emotion(s).	Write your stuck point related to the situation in Section A. Rate your belief in this stuck point from 0 to 100%. (How strongly do you believe this thought?)	Specify your emotion(s) (sad, angry, etc.) and rate how strongly you feel each emotion from 0 to 100%.	Use the **exploring questions** to examine your automatic thought from Section B. Consider whether the thought is balanced and factual or extreme.	Use the **thinking patterns** to decide whether this is one of the patterns and explain why.	What else can you say instead of the thought in Section B? How else can you interpret the event instead of this thought? Rate your belief in the alternative thought(s) from 0 to 100%.
			Evidence against?	Jumping to conclusions:	
			What information is not included?	Ignoring important parts:	
			All or none? Extreme?	Oversimplifying/overgeneralizing:	
			Focused on just one piece of the event?		
			Questionable source of information?	Mind reading:	**G. Re-rate old stuck point** Re-rate how much you now believe the stuck point in Section B from 0 to 100%.
			Confusing possible with definite?		
			Based on feelings or facts?	Emotional reasoning:	**H. Emotion(s)** Now what do you feel? Rate from 0 to 100%.

Alternative Thoughts Worksheet

A. Situation	B. Stuck point	D. Exploring thoughts	E. Thinking patterns	F. Alternative thought(s)
Describe the event leading to the stuck point or unpleasant emotion(s).	Write your stuck point related to the situation in Section A. Rate your belief in this stuck point from 0 to 100%. (How strongly do you believe this thought?)	Use the **exploring questions** to examine your automatic thought from Section B. Consider whether the thought is balanced and factual or extreme.	Use the **thinking patterns** to decide whether this is one of the patterns and explain why.	What else can you say instead of the thought in Section B? How else can you interpret the event instead of this thought? Rate your belief in the alternative thought(s) from 0 to 100%.
		Evidence against?	Jumping to conclusions:	
		What information is not included?	Ignoring important parts:	
		All or none? Extreme?	Oversimplifying/overgeneralizing:	
		Focused on just one piece of the event?		
		Questionable source of information?	Mind reading:	**G. Re-rate old stuck point**
		Confusing possible with definite?		Re-rate how much you now believe the stuck point in Section B from 0 to 100%.
	C. Emotion(s) Specify your emotion(s) (sad, angry, etc.) and rate how strongly you feel each emotion from 0 to 100%.	Based on feelings or facts?	Emotional reasoning:	**H. Emotion(s)** Now what do you feel? Rate from 0 to 100%.

Alternative Thoughts Worksheet

A. Situation	B. Stuck point	D. Exploring thoughts	E. Thinking patterns	F. Alternative thought(s)
Describe the event leading to the stuck point or unpleasant emotion(s).	Write your stuck point related to the situation in Section A. Rate your belief in this stuck point from 0 to 100%. (How strongly do you believe this thought?)	Use the **exploring questions** to examine your automatic thought from Section B. Consider whether the thought is balanced and factual or extreme.	Use the **thinking patterns** to decide whether this is one of the patterns and explain why.	What else can you say instead of the thought in Section B? How else can you interpret the event instead of this thought? Rate your belief in the alternative thought(s) from 0 to 100%.
		Evidence against?	Jumping to conclusions:	
		What information is not included?	Ignoring important parts:	
		All or none? Extreme?	Oversimplifying/overgeneralizing:	
		Focused on just one piece of the event?		
	C. Emotion(s) Specify your emotion(s) (sad, angry, etc.) and rate how strongly you feel each emotion from 0 to 100%.	Questionable source of information?	Mind reading:	**G. Re-rate old stuck point** Re-rate how much you now believe the stuck point in Section B from 0 to 100%.
		Confusing possible with definite?		
		Based on feelings or facts?	Emotional reasoning:	**H. Emotion(s)** Now what do you feel? Rate from 0 to 100%.

From *Getting Unstuck from PTSD* by Patricia A. Resick, Shannon Wiltsey Stirman, and Stefanie T. LoSavio. Copyright © 2023 The Guilford Press. Purchasers of this book can photocopy and/or download additional copies of this worksheet at www.guilford.com/resick2-forms for personal use or use with clients; see copyright page for details.

(PTSD Checklist)

Complete the PTSD Checklist to track your symptoms as you complete this book. Be sure to complete this measure on the same index event each time. When the instructions and questions refer to a "stressful experience," remember that that is your index event—the worst event that you are working on first.

Write in here the trauma that you are working on first: _____

Complete this PTSD Checklist with reference to that event.

Instructions: Below is a list of problems that people sometimes have in response to a very stressful experience. Please read each problem carefully, and then circle one of the numbers to the right to indicate how much you have been bothered by that problem *in the past week*.

In the past week, how much were you bothered by:	Not at all	A little bit	Mod- erately	Quite a bit	Extremely
1. Repeated, disturbing, and unwanted memories of the stressful experience?	0	1	2	3	4
2. Repeated, disturbing dreams of the stressful experience?	0	1	2	3	4
3. Suddenly feeling or acting as if the stressful experience were actually happening again (*as if you were actually back there reliving it*)?	0	1	2	3	4
4. Feeling very upset when something reminded you of the stressful experience?	0	1	2	3	4
5. Having strong physical reactions when something reminded you of the stressful experience (*for example, heart pounding, trouble breathing, sweating*)?	0	1	2	3	4
6. Avoiding memories, thoughts, or feelings related to the stressful experience?	0	1	2	3	4
7. Avoiding external reminders of the stressful experience (*for example, people, places, conversations, activities, objects, or situations*)?	0	1	2	3	4
8. Trouble remembering important parts of the stressful experience (not due to head injury or substances)?	0	1	2	3	4
9. Having strong negative beliefs about yourself, other people, or the world (*for example, having thoughts such as I am bad, There is something seriously wrong with me, No one can be trusted, or The world is completely dangerous*)?	0	1	2	3	4
10. Blaming yourself or someone else (who didn't intend the outcome) for the stressful experience or what happened after it?	0	1	2	3	4
11. Having strong negative feelings, such as fear, horror, anger, guilt, or shame?	0	1	2	3	4
12. Loss of interest in activities that you used to enjoy?	0	1	2	3	4
13. Feeling distant or cut off from other people?	0	1	2	3	4
14. Trouble experiencing positive feelings (*for example, being unable to feel happiness or have loving feelings for people close to you*)?	0	1	2	3	4
15. Irritable behavior, angry outbursts, or acting aggressively?	0	1	2	3	4
16. Taking too many risks or doing things that could cause you harm?	0	1	2	3	4
17. Being "super alert" or watchful or on guard?	0	1	2	3	4
18. Feeling jumpy or easily startled?	0	1	2	3	4
19. Having difficulty concentrating?	0	1	2	3	4
20. Trouble falling or staying asleep?	0	1	2	3	4

Add up the total and write it here: _____

From *PTSD Checklist for DSM-5 (PCL-5)* by Weathers, Litz, Keane, Palmieri, Marx, and Schnurr (2013). Available from the National Center for PTSD at *www.ptsd.va.gov*; in the public domain. Reprinted in *Getting Unstuck from PTSD* (Guilford Press, 2023). Purchasers of this book can photocopy and/or download additional copies of this worksheet at *www.guilford.com/resick2-forms* for personal use or use with clients; see copyright page for details.

15

Intimacy

The final theme is intimacy. Intimacy does not just mean physical and sexual intimacy—it means a close familiarity. This includes a number of dimensions, such as friendship and emotional intimacy with others, and self-intimacy, self-awareness, and trust with yourself in terms of your wants, needs, and sense of who you are. PTSD can change the way you relate to and interact with yourself and others, and having fully realized, healthy relationships with yourself and others can take some intentional, focused work.

Intimacy with others includes the full range of relationships from acquaintanceships, friendships, family relationships, and up to and including having a partner with a deep bond and sexual intimacy. Relationships take a long time to develop, so the goal of this chapter is to work on stuck points that have interfered with your being able to enrich the quality of relationships or develop new ones. Remember from Chapter 12 on trust that you don't have to trust someone in every possible way to have them in your life.

You may have avoided intimate relationships for quite some time because of your beliefs about yourself and others that resulted from the traumatic event. Now that you've been working through issues of trust, power and control, and esteem, you have the opportunity to consider stuck points that have kept you from getting close to people. You may notice stuck points that led you to pull back from friendships or from close relationships, like "If I get too close, people will hurt me" or "Nobody will accept me." Look out for stuck points like these and remember to use what you learned about trust as you begin moving toward closer relationships. Some people will be accepting and may have had their own traumatic or difficult experiences that will actually help them relate to you and understand you when you express your needs, hopes, fears, and concerns. Others may want to try to understand and may be open to feedback from you as they respond to your efforts to get closer. And if people are not able or willing to respond to your efforts to be closer in ways that are healthy for you, that's information that they may not be the healthiest people to get close to, but perhaps they can be more casual friends or acquaintances, or family members that you have more limited contact with. As you learned in the trust chapter, you do not need to trust someone in every possible way before allowing them into your life, and there are more limited ways to have people in your life. Think about the potential for friendships and how casual or close you want to be.

If you are married or in a committed romantic relationship and your relationship is rocky, your partner may not know how to react to the changes you've been making as you complete this process. You may want to consider couple or family therapy. There are also couple-based PTSD treatments, including an online course called Couple HOPES (*www. couplehopes.com*) that can help. Sometimes if you have had PTSD for a long time and felt unable to do certain activities or go certain places, your partner may have taken on a care-giver role. As you no longer need this, your partner may feel that they lost an important function in your relationship. You'll want to work on open communication and perhaps renegotiate tasks and activities. They may also have gotten used to going out and doing things without you, and you may need to work together to reintegrate into each other's lives in a different way. If the trauma that you experienced was a sexual assault or abuse, you may also have stuck points about sexual intimacy that you need to examine.

Stuck points that are specific to sexual relationships may include "Sex is unsafe" or "If I am physically intimate with someone, they will exploit me." It can really feel like a risk to become sexually intimate. Remember that this is not something that you need to rush. It takes time to build trust and to develop emotional closeness, which might be important elements for you to establish first if you have been avoiding sexual intimacy. You can take your time to see how partners or potential partners will react as you share any concerns you have about physical intimacy. If they don't react in a way that is comfortable for you, that's important evidence about whether they are the right partner for you at this time in your life.

Self-intimacy is more than self-esteem. It's the ability to really know and accept yourself, to soothe and care for yourself without relying on external or perhaps destructive behaviors (but using the worksheets would be a healthy method!). It's about becoming comfortable in your own skin, with who you are, and accepting yourself as you are. That includes being able to be alone without being lonely. Self-intimacy is knowing what your values and tastes are. It's being comfortable understanding your limits and boundaries and not being afraid to maintain them in order to be true to and to honor yourself. Doing something nice or worthwhile for yourself every day is a way to find out what you enjoy doing and perhaps haven't done because of the aftermath of traumatic events.

Self-intimacy is deciding how you want to spend your time and what your goals are for the future. This is an ongoing process, but you might look around at other people your own age and see what they're doing with their lives and free time, such as deciding on the path they want to take with their career or education; finding hobbies or spiritual activities that they find fulfilling; or deciding whether they want their lives to include a partner, children, or pets. If you are a young adult, your age-mates are also deciding who they want to be and may experiment with different careers or locations. Think of yourself as "graduating" from your PTSD and moving on to a different chapter in your life. If you are older, your age-mates might be going through a change of identity as they retire and decide how they want to spend their time and where they want to do that. You could think of yourself as "retiring" from your PTSD. Even midlife carries changes as people's bodies, interests, relationships, and activities change. Other people may have children out of the home now and are suddenly free to engage in new interests, or they may have more responsibilities as a caregiver for their parents. In other words, self-intimacy is the process of coming to know yourself again without PTSD, and it will extend well beyond the time you spend going through this book and into the rest of your life. But remember, being comfortable with yourself also means accepting yourself and your interests even if they differ from those that other people have. You may choose to spend some time without being in a romantic relationship. You may choose a path for yourself that isn't like the one that others have chosen. That's OK, too—just make sure that your decisions are driven by your sense of who you are and what you want and not by stuck points and PTSD.

> Margaret had a history of sexual trauma and also experienced intimate partner violence. After she left her abusive marriage and started working on her PTSD, she began to work on the self-blame around the abuse ("I should have left sooner. It's my fault because I stayed"), her sense of trust of others, and trusting herself when she saw red flags in other relationships. She worked on addressing her stuck points around power and control so that she could feel more confident in setting boundaries, and she learned to reengage with friends and family members, gradually sharing more about her trauma history with people who supported her. She noticed, though, that she continued to hold back from forming romantic relationships. She would stop responding to men who showed interest in her, even though she realized she wanted to eventually share her life with someone. She identified several stuck points that kept her from exploring or pursuing romantic relationships, including "All he wants is sex" and "I'm not capable of having healthy relationships." She used the worksheets to examine the evidence for these beliefs. She also realized that sometimes she didn't have enough information to really know. She began to slowly form relationships with men, beginning with things like talking over coffee, spending time together in groups, and taking walks together. She learned that some men were willing to, and even wanted to, take their time to get to know her. This was evidence against the belief that men only wanted sex. She remembered what she learned about trust and took her time in disclosing private information that made her feel vulnerable, only after she had evidence that she could trust them with other information. She also learned to set boundaries when men wanted to move faster than she wished to and discovered that she could tolerate it when she needed to end relationships that didn't feel like they were progressing in a healthy or comfortable way. Over time, she came to see that she was, in fact, able to form healthy relationships. The fact that she had not been in a healthy relationship in the past didn't mean she couldn't use her developing skills to form the relationships she wanted in the future.

Resolving stuck points about intimacy is just the beginning of developing a better relationship with yourself and others. As with esteem, you may need a lot of practice with the Alternative Thoughts Worksheets (see pages 255–261) and with your actions in the world to change years of avoiding people and avoiding yourself. Don't worry if you have some setbacks. They are a part of life, and each one gives you an opportunity to learn more about yourself, refine your response, and ultimately become stronger and more confident about who you are. You have lived through a lot, and you have shown resilience and strength by facing your PTSD. Now you can work to build the life that you want for yourself, knowing that you can face hard things and overcome them and that you have the tools to keep moving forward.

☑ Key Points on the Topic of Intimacy

Consider how the trauma impacted your sense of intimacy with self and others. Did it confirm beliefs your already held? Or did it lead you to question your ability to be intimate with others, or your sense of self-intimacy?

Beliefs Related to Self

How you cope with the trauma and memories is influenced by your sense of self-intimacy. Self-intimacy is the ability to be alone without feeling lonely or empty. When you can soothe yourself and cope with stress without feeling completely dependent on others, that's a sign of self-intimacy too. While it's important to feel supported and not isolate, it's also important to be able to navigate the world with independence, so that you can be in relationships that are not overly dependent and don't feel you have no choice but to be in an unhealthy relationship so that you aren't alone.

➲ If you had stable and positive self-intimacy and the trauma or its aftermath conflicted with your earlier beliefs (for example, if you had trouble coping in the aftermath), it may have left you feeling anxious or overwhelmed. Traumas are not the same as everyday stressors, and it makes sense that you didn't cope in the same way you did with other life events.

➲ If you had previous experiences that led you to believe you couldn't cope with life events, or if you didn't have good examples from the adults in your life when you were growing up, you may have reacted to the trauma with beliefs that you were unable to comfort or take care of yourself. This can lead to avoidance of trauma reminders.

A lower sense of self-intimacy can lead to a fear of being alone, difficulty comforting or soothing yourself, a feeling of inner emptiness, and forming needy or demanding relationships. You may also find yourself looking outside yourself for comfort through food, drugs or alcohol, medications, spending money, or sex.

Pretrauma belief	Posttrauma stuck points	Possible balanced/alternative thoughts
I can cope when stressful things happen.	I am helpless and unable to deal with what happened.	What happened wasn't just an everyday stressor. It was really terrible, and everyone has a hard time after something like this.
		My feelings will fade over time.
		I'm learning skills and letting myself process the trauma now, and that will help.

Pretrauma belief	Posttrauma stuck points	Possible balanced/alternative thoughts
I can't handle it when bad things happen.	I need to [drink/ use drugs/not be alone/overeat/ shop/etc.] to feel better.	Doing those things only helps in the short term, and they leave me with other problems. I can tolerate more than I think I can. If I let myself feel these things and if I use my coping skills, I can get through difficult times—even if it's hard.
I have a sense of who I am.	I don't know who I am anymore.	I can listen to myself about my preferences, wants, needs, and feelings and discover or rediscover my sense of self over time.

Intimacy Related to Others

Connection, closeness, and intimacy are basic human needs. Our ability to be intimately connected with people can be damaged by hurtful, insensitive, or unempathetic behavior from others. Intimacy can refer to both emotional and physical intimacy. Emotional intimacy can occur with friends, family, or romantic partners.

- ⊃ If you had healthy intimate relationships before the traumatic event, the trauma may have left you believing you could never be intimate with others again, especially if you were harmed by someone you knew or trusted. You may also have found that your beliefs about intimacy changed if people you trusted were unsupportive, rejected you, or treated you differently after the trauma.

- ⊃ If you had a history of unhealthy or abusive relationships, the trauma may have confirmed your negative beliefs about intimacy.

Difficulties with intimacy can leave you feeling lonely, isolated, empty, and disconnected, even in healthy and loving relationships.

Pretrauma belief	Posttrauma stuck points	Possible balanced/alternative thoughts
I can be close with people I care about without getting hurt.	If I get too close, people will hurt me.	Even though I was hurt in a relationship, it doesn't mean that it's not possible to have a healthy relationship. I can take it slow, ask for what I need, and develop something healthy. I can also leave if I learn that the other person does not treat me well.

Pretrauma belief	Posttrauma stuck points	Possible balanced/alternative thoughts
I am capable of having healthy relationships.	If a relationship fails, it's my fault.	It takes two to have a healthy relationship. I can try hard and communicate, but the other person has to meet me halfway.
If a relationship doesn't work out, it's my fault.	I am too broken or damaged to have a healthy relationship.	The trauma doesn't define me. I have many things to offer in a relationship. People who care about me will understand if I need to take it slow and build trust. People who are unwilling to do that are showing me that they are not the right partner for me.
It's not safe to get close to people.	I need to remain alone.	My past experiences have been hard, but it doesn't mean that healthy relationships aren't possible. It may take me some time to trust and figure out who is safe to open up to, but it may be worth the risk to feel less lonely and more connected.
Relationships can be healthy.	I will be hurt or exploited in relationships.	It's possible to be in a healthy relationship. And even if one doesn't work out, I can learn from it and move forward alone or in another relationship.

▶▶ To watch a video to review what you just read here about intimacy, go to the CPT Whiteboard Video Library (*http://cptforptsd.com/cpt-resources*) and watch the videos called *Self-Intimacy* and *Intimacy Related to Others.*

 PRACTICE ASSIGNMENT

Look over your Stuck Point Log on page 56 to pick out the stuck points that are concerned with self- or other-intimacy. If you have issues with self- or other-intimacy, complete Alternative Thoughts Worksheets on them (see pages 255–261). Also notice whether you still have any stuck points about why the trauma happened that are related to intimacy, such as "The trauma happened because I let that person in." If so, do those first.

Also, don't forget to keep giving and receiving compliments and doing nice and worthwhile things for yourself! Remember, these are things you want to integrate into your everyday life now. Work on any stuck points that make it difficult to do them.

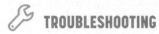 **TROUBLESHOOTING**

I'm still stuck. I'm having a hard time letting go of my intimacy beliefs.

If you're having a hard time letting go of your intimacy beliefs like "If I let someone in, they will hurt me," consider whether you still have any related *intimacy beliefs about why your traumatic event occurred,* and if so, do those first. For example, if you're still thinking "The trauma happened because I let that person in," it's no surprise you are worried about letting others in. However, reconsider the facts of the trauma. Did the trauma happen because you let someone in, or did it happen because that person chose to hurt you? Go back and do an Alternative Thoughts Worksheet on the intimacy stuck point about why the trauma happened. Then see if you can make more progress on the more general stuck points about intimacy.

I can't stop having images when I try to be physically intimate. It disgusts me.

Remember that sexual abuse and sexual assault are crimes and have *nothing* to do with sexual intimacy. Have you talked to your partner about the struggles you are having with physical intimacy? Do they even know what happened to you? It's amazing how many people haven't told their partners about their experiences. If your partner has shown themselves to be trustworthy with your personal information and emotions, you may want to tell them why intimacy is difficult for you. Remember, you can tell them that you experienced sexual assault without going into details that you aren't comfortable sharing. If they are surprised you never told them this before, you can explain why you didn't tell them (shame, embarrassment) and that it's part of your PTSD and not anything about your partner. You may want to seek out some form of therapy (couple or sex therapy), but you could try to do some Alternative Thoughts Worksheets first to make sure that you don't have general stuck points about sex and intimacy. It can be tougher if you were raped by a former partner, someone you ideally should have been able to trust with your body and to care for you. You can ask your partner if you could take it slow for a bit while you work on your stuck points. Try just kissing or touching first. Keep your eyes open and focus on where you are in the moment. Focus on the person you are with and remember that this is someone different from the person who hurt you. If you freeze or have a flashback, ask to stop for a moment so that you can calm down and focus on the present moment. Talk about this in advance so your partner isn't startled by it, and tell them how they can support you in situations like this. If your partner can't do this for you, it's a sign you should strongly consider couple treatment or think about whether this is the partner you want to continue with.

Alternative Thoughts Worksheet

A. Situation	B. Stuck point	D. Exploring thoughts	E. Thinking patterns	F. Alternative thought(s)
Describe the event leading to the stuck point or unpleasant emotion(s).	Write your stuck point related to the situation in Section A. Rate your belief in this stuck point from 0 to 100%. (How strongly do you believe this thought?)	Use the **exploring questions** to examine your automatic thought from Section B. Consider whether the thought is balanced and factual or extreme.	Use the **thinking patterns** to decide whether this is one of the patterns and explain why.	What else can you say instead of the thought in Section B? How else can you interpret the event instead of this thought? Rate your belief in the alternative thought(s) from 0 to 100%.
		Evidence against?	Jumping to conclusions:	
		What information is not included?	Ignoring important parts:	
		All or none? Extreme?		
		Focused on just one piece of the event?	Oversimplifying/overgeneralizing:	
		Questionable source of information?	Mind reading:	G. Re-rate old stuck point Re-rate how much you now believe the stuck point in Section B from 0 to 100%.
		Confusing possible with definite?		
	C. Emotion(s) Specify your emotion(s) (sad, angry, etc.) and rate how strongly you feel each emotion from 0 to 100%.	Based on feelings or facts?	Emotional reasoning:	**H. Emotion(s)** Now what do you feel? Rate from 0 to 100%.

Alternative Thoughts Worksheet

A. Situation	B. Stuck point	C. Emotion(s)	D. Exploring thoughts	E. Thinking patterns	F. Alternative thought(s)
Describe the event leading to the stuck point or unpleasant emotion(s).	Write your stuck point related to the situation in Section A. Rate your belief in this stuck point from 0 to 100%. (How strongly do you believe this thought?)		Use the **exploring questions** to examine your automatic thought from Section B. Consider whether the thought is balanced and factual or extreme.	Use the **thinking patterns** to decide whether this is one of the patterns and explain why.	What else can you say instead of the thought in Section B? How else can you interpret the event instead of this thought? Rate your belief in the alternative thought(s) from 0 to 100%.
			Evidence against?	Jumping to conclusions:	
			What information is not included?	Ignoring important parts:	
			All or none? Extreme?		
			Focused on just one piece of the event?	Oversimplifying/overgeneralizing:	
		C. Emotion(s) Specify your emotion(s) (sad, angry, etc.) and rate how strongly you feel each emotion from 0 to 100%.	Questionable source of information?	Mind reading:	**G. Re-rate old stuck point** Re-rate how much you now believe the stuck point in Section B from 0 to 100%.
			Confusing possible with definite?		
			Based on feelings or facts?	Emotional reasoning:	**H. Emotion(s)** Now what do you feel? Rate from 0 to 100%.

Alternative Thoughts Worksheet

A. Situation	B. Stuck point	C. Emotion(s)	D. Exploring thoughts	E. Thinking patterns	F. Alternative thought(s)	G. Re-rate old stuck point	H. Emotion(s)
Describe the event leading to the stuck point or unpleasant emotion(s).	Write your stuck point related to the situation in Section A. Rate your belief in this stuck point from 0 to 100%. (How strongly do you believe this thought?)	Specify your emotion(s) (sad, angry, etc.) and rate how strongly you feel each emotion from 0 to 100%.	Use the **exploring questions** to examine your automatic thought from Section B. Consider whether the thought is balanced and factual or extreme.	Use the **thinking patterns** to decide whether this is one of the patterns and explain why.	What else can you say instead of the thought in Section B? How else can you interpret the event instead of this thought? Rate your belief in the alternative thought(s) from 0 to 100%.	Re-rate how much you now believe the stuck point in Section B from 0 to 100%.	Now what do you feel? Rate from 0 to 100%.
			Evidence against?	Jumping to conclusions:			
			What information is not included?	Ignoring important parts:			
			All or none? Extreme?				
			Focused on just one piece of the event?	Oversimplifying/overgeneralizing:			
			Questionable source of information?	Mind reading:			
			Confusing possible with definite?				
			Based on feelings or facts?	Emotional reasoning:			

Alternative Thoughts Worksheet

A. Situation	B. Stuck point	C. Emotion(s)	D. Exploring thoughts	E. Thinking patterns	F. Alternative thought(s)
Describe the event leading to the stuck point or unpleasant emotion(s).	Write your stuck point related to the situation in Section A. Rate your belief in this stuck point from 0 to 100%. (How strongly do you believe this thought?)	Specify your emotion(s) (sad, angry, etc.) and rate how strongly you feel each emotion from 0 to 100%.	Use the **exploring questions** to examine your automatic thought from Section B. Consider whether the thought is balanced and factual or extreme.	Use the **thinking patterns** to decide whether this is one of the patterns and explain why.	What else can you say instead of the thought in Section B? How else can you interpret the event instead of this thought? Rate your belief in the alternative thought(s) from 0 to 100%.
			Evidence against?	Jumping to conclusions:	
			What information is not included?	Ignoring important parts:	
			All or none? Extreme?		
			Focused on just one piece of the event?	Oversimplifying/overgeneralizing:	
			Questionable source of information?	Mind reading:	G. Re-rate old stuck point
			Confusing possible with definite?		Re-rate how much you now believe the stuck point in Section B from 0 to 100%.
			Based on feelings or facts?	Emotional reasoning:	
					H. Emotion(s) Now what do you feel? Rate from 0 to 100%.

From *Getting Unstuck from PTSD* by Patricia A. Resick, Shannon Wiltsey Stirman, and Stefanie T. LoSavio. Copyright © 2023 The Guilford Press. Purchasers of this book can photocopy and/or download additional copies of this worksheet at www.guilford.com/resick2-forms for personal use or use with clients; see copyright page for details.

Alternative Thoughts Worksheet

A. Situation	B. Stuck point	D. Exploring thoughts	E. Thinking patterns	F. Alternative thought(s)
Describe the event leading to the stuck point or unpleasant emotion(s).	Write your stuck point related to the situation in Section A. Rate your belief in this stuck point from 0 to 100%. (How strongly do you believe this thought?)	Use the **exploring questions** to examine your automatic thought from Section B. Consider whether the thought is balanced and factual or extreme.	Use the **thinking patterns** to decide whether this is one of the patterns and explain why.	What else can you say instead of the thought in Section B? How else can you interpret the event instead of this thought? Rate your belief in the alternative thought(s) from 0 to 100%.
		Evidence against?	Jumping to conclusions:	
		What information is not included?	Ignoring important parts:	
		All or none? Extreme?		
		Focused on just one piece of the event?	Oversimplifying/overgeneralizing:	
	C. Emotion(s) Specify your emotion(s) (sad, angry, etc.) and rate how strongly you feel each emotion from 0 to 100%.	Questionable source of information?	Mind reading:	**G. Re-rate old stuck point** Re-rate how much you now believe the stuck point in Section B from 0 to 100%.
		Confusing possible with definite?		
		Based on feelings or facts?	Emotional reasoning:	**H. Emotion(s)** Now what do you feel? Rate from 0 to 100%.

From *Getting Unstuck from PTSD* by Patricia A. Resick, Shannon Wiltsey Stirman, and Stefanie T. LoSavio. Copyright © 2023 The Guilford Press. Purchasers of this book can photocopy and/or download additional copies of this worksheet at www.guilford.com/resick2-forms for personal use or use with clients; see copyright page for details.

Alternative Thoughts Worksheet

A. Situation	B. Stuck point	C. Emotion(s)	D. Exploring thoughts	E. Thinking patterns	F. Alternative thought(s)
Describe the event leading to the stuck point or unpleasant emotion(s).	Write your stuck point related to the situation in Section A. Rate your belief in this stuck point from 0 to 100%. (How strongly do you believe this thought?)	Specify your emotion(s) (sad, angry, etc.) and rate how strongly you feel each emotion from 0 to 100%.	Use the **exploring questions** to examine your automatic thought from Section B. Consider whether the thought is balanced and factual or extreme.	Use the **thinking patterns** to decide whether this is one of the patterns and explain why.	What else can you say instead of the thought in Section B? How else can you interpret the event instead of this thought? Rate your belief in the alternative thought(s) from 0 to 100%.
			Evidence against?	Jumping to conclusions:	
			What information is not included?	Ignoring important parts:	
			All or none? Extreme?		
			Focused on just one piece of the event?	Oversimplifying/overgeneralizing:	
			Questionable source of information?	Mind reading:	G. Re-rate old stuck point: Re-rate how much you now believe the stuck point in Section B from 0 to 100%.
			Confusing possible with definite?		
			Based on feelings or facts?	Emotional reasoning:	H. Emotion(s): Now what do you feel? Rate from 0 to 100%.

Alternative Thoughts Worksheet

A. Situation	B. Stuck point	C. Emotion(s)	D. Exploring thoughts	E. Thinking patterns	F. Alternative thought(s)	G. Re-rate old stuck point	H. Emotion(s)
Describe the event leading to the stuck point or unpleasant emotion(s).	Write your stuck point related to the situation in Section A. Rate your belief in this stuck point from 0 to 100%. (How strongly do you believe this thought?)	Specify your emotion(s) (sad, angry, etc.) and rate how strongly you feel each emotion from 0 to 100%.	Use the **exploring questions** to examine your automatic thought from Section B. Consider whether the thought is balanced and factual or extreme. Evidence against? What information is not included? All or none? Extreme? Focused on just one piece of the event? Questionable source of information? Confusing possible with definite? Based on feelings or facts?	Use the **thinking patterns** to decide whether this is one of the patterns and explain why. Jumping to conclusions: Ignoring important parts: Oversimplifying/overgeneralizing: Mind reading: Emotional reasoning:	What else can you say instead of the thought in Section B? How else can you interpret the event instead of this thought? Rate your belief in the alternative thought(s) from 0 to 100%.	Re-rate how much you now believe the stuck point in Section B from 0 to 100%.	Now what do you feel? Rate from 0 to 100%.

I still don't let myself feel emotions.

First, remember to differentiate between natural and manufactured emotions. You don't have to continue to feel the manufactured emotions, which are based on your stuck points. Doing worksheets on them can help them diminish or change. Often the emotions that people with PTSD avoid are natural emotions, like sadness that the trauma happened or anger at a perpetrator. If you are avoiding feeling natural emotions, there may be a stuck point about emotions in general or perhaps one specific emotion. What are you thinking will happen if you feel your emotions? Is your stuck point that they'll make you weak or vulnerable? Watch sports figures at a championship game or at the Olympics and you'll see amazingly strong people crying with sadness or happiness. Nothing bad happens to them, and no one calls them wimps. Are you afraid that if you start to feel an emotion it will never stop? Is that even possible? At some point you would be so worn out that you would fall asleep or begin to calm down. You might have a headache or a runny nose, but no catastrophe happens from feeling emotions. Behaviors get people into trouble, not emotions. Try to just sit there and feel them. Think of shaking up a bottle of soda and then opening the lid. If you immediately put the lid back on, the carbonation is still there and feels quite explosive. However, if you hold it over the sink, shake it up, and open the lid, there will be a burst of liquid and then it will calm down. Then, no matter how much you shake it, you won't see that many more bubbles (emotions) again. What other stuck points might you have about allowing yourself to feel your emotions?

How do I figure out who I am without my PTSD?

That's a good question that many people have to explore after PTSD. If they have lived in avoidance for many years, some people lose touch with what their values are and what activities they enjoy, and they may have also lost touch with friends. It's a good time to take stock and decide what's important to you and what's not so important. It may be a good time to try out new things to see if you might discover some new interests. You may be able to reconnect with people again even after many years. You aren't going to go back to the person you were when the traumatic events started because even if they hadn't happened, you would have changed and grown by now. Don't set a goal to be the person you used to be. Set a goal to be the person you would like to become. Consider what developmental tasks people your own age are taking on. Start by focusing on events outside of yourself. Read about things you're interested in—talk to other people about their lives. Join a group or take a class to get some ideas.

When should I tell someone about my history?

Telling someone about your trauma history is a matter of personal choice and depends on how close you are with that person. Acquaintances with whom you have a superficial relationship that concerns an activity or work don't need to know. If you are moving into friendship with someone and they disclose something personal about themselves, you might take a chance and tell them that you have a trauma history, without going into details. You wouldn't typically want to tell someone on a first date that you were raped. That is just too much information, especially if neither of you has decided whether you want it to be more than one date. Even if you think you should disclose it to explain why you want to limit physical intimacy, remember that you don't need to justify your boundaries. Consider why you want to tell someone you don't know well. Is it to see how they react in order to determine whether you can trust them? Be careful not to use your trauma history as a test. No one likes pop quizzes, so don't surprise them with information about yourself just to see what their reaction will be. It's not fair to either of you. In an ongoing relationship, there will come a point when you both let each other into your histories, and that might be an appropriate time. Once you are more securely in a relationship and have already observed a person be supportive in response to other details about you, you might share some of the details of your trauma, but you are never required to give all of the details of any specific event. How much to tell is a very personal decision.

When do you go from acquaintance to friend?

Going from acquaintance to friend is a mutual and usually unspoken decision. It usually happens gradually if you like each other, feel better (rather than worse) when being with that person, and enjoy spending time together. Friendships come out of equal desire to spend time or company with each other (even if just by text message) and are only fifty percent your decision. Friendships can ebb and flow, so don't take it personally if you lose touch with some people while you gain others. Tastes and goals change over the course of a lifetime, and friendships can be that way too. Some friendships can pick up right where they left off even if you haven't seen someone for a long time because you have a base of caring and respect for each other. Some will fade out naturally because of work or family obligations or distance that makes seeing each other difficult. Most people have very few people in their lives they consider close friends but many more who are acquaintances.

* * *

You've come a long way! Take a moment to complete the PTSD Checklist to assess your current symptom level.

Planning for the Conclusion of CPT

Many people complete CPT after they work through the chapter on intimacy. If you have met your goals and worked through your main stuck points, you'll graduate at the next chapter. Keep in mind that you don't have to resolve all of your stuck points or have "no" symptoms to move forward. However, you may be ready to graduate if you have addressed many of the stuck points that were keeping you stuck in PTSD, have reduced your symptoms (ideally a score of 19 or below on the PTSD Checklist), and have the skills to continue working on any remaining issues. If you are ready to wrap up your work, go to the final chapter to review your progress and plan for the future.

(PTSD Checklist)

Complete the PTSD Checklist to track your symptoms as you complete this book. Be sure to complete this measure on the same index event each time. When the instructions and questions refer to a "stressful experience," remember that that is your index event—the worst event that you are working on first.

Write in here the trauma that you are working on first: _____

Complete this PTSD Checklist with reference to that event.

Instructions: Below is a list of problems that people sometimes have in response to a very stressful experience. Please read each problem carefully, and then circle one of the numbers to the right to indicate how much you have been bothered by that problem *in the past week*.

In the past week, how much were you bothered by:	Not at all	A little bit	Mod-erately	Quite a bit	Extremely
1. Repeated, disturbing, and unwanted memories of the stressful experience?	0	1	2	3	4
2. Repeated, disturbing dreams of the stressful experience?	0	1	2	3	4
3. Suddenly feeling or acting as if the stressful experience were actually happening again (*as if you were actually back there reliving it*)?	0	1	2	3	4
4. Feeling very upset when something reminded you of the stressful experience?	0	1	2	3	4
5. Having strong physical reactions when something reminded you of the stressful experience (*for example, heart pounding, trouble breathing, sweating*)?	0	1	2	3	4
6. Avoiding memories, thoughts, or feelings related to the stressful experience?	0	1	2	3	4
7. Avoiding external reminders of the stressful experience (*for example, people, places, conversations, activities, objects, or situations*)?	0	1	2	3	4
8. Trouble remembering important parts of the stressful experience (not due to head injury or substances)?	0	1	2	3	4
9. Having strong negative beliefs about yourself, other people, or the world (*for example, having thoughts such as I am bad, There is something seriously wrong with me, No one can be trusted, or The world is completely dangerous*)?	0	1	2	3	4
10. Blaming yourself or someone else (who didn't intend the outcome) for the stressful experience or what happened after it?	0	1	2	3	4
11. Having strong negative feelings, such as fear, horror, anger, guilt, or shame?	0	1	2	3	4
12. Loss of interest in activities that you used to enjoy?	0	1	2	3	4
13. Feeling distant or cut off from other people?	0	1	2	3	4
14. Trouble experiencing positive feelings (*for example, being unable to feel happiness or have loving feelings for people close to you*)?	0	1	2	3	4
15. Irritable behavior, angry outbursts, or acting aggressively?	0	1	2	3	4
16. Taking too many risks or doing things that could cause you harm?	0	1	2	3	4
17. Being "super alert" or watchful or on guard?	0	1	2	3	4
18. Feeling jumpy or easily startled?	0	1	2	3	4
19. Having difficulty concentrating?	0	1	2	3	4
20. Trouble falling or staying asleep?	0	1	2	3	4

Add up the total and write it here: _____

Continuing Your Work

Alternatively, you may choose to continue practicing the CPT skills with worksheets a while longer. If you are still having significant PTSD symptoms and have specific goals for continuing (such as a few more key stuck points to address), you can continue for as long as you need. There are no new topics, so you'll just continue to work with your Stuck Point Log and worksheets. If you've decided that it would be helpful to extend your work, make a plan for which stuck points you'll work on as you continue. You may want to revisit earlier topics that were not completely resolved or work on stuck points about a different traumatic event.

It can help to go through your Stuck Point Log and cross off any stuck points that you no longer believe. The stuck points that remain are the ones you still need to work on. In the Appendix, you will find a blank Stuck Point Log for Remaining Stuck Points that you can use to write down the stuck points you want to continue working on. Continue to use the worksheets to explore those thoughts. Extra Alternative Thoughts Worksheets can be found on pages 255–261.

If you've already tried examining some of your remaining stuck points and they still feel stuck, you might try wording the stuck points in different ways (for example, "If I hadn't done _____, I would have prevented the event" or "If only I had done _____, it never would have happened"). Sometimes changing the stuck point around a little bit will help you see it from different angles. Ask yourself what you mean by the stuck point.

You can also ask yourself some questions if you are particularly stuck, such as:

- How would you feel if you let go of that belief?
- Are you using this stuck point to protect against a scarier idea (for example, "If I couldn't have prevented the event, then there might be other events in the future I won't be able to prevent")?
- Is there a stuck point that keeps you from embracing recovery like "If I start to recover, it will mean the traumatic event didn't matter"?
- Is there a core belief that is holding this stuck point in place, such as "Everything is always my fault" or "The world is completely dangerous"? If you always react as though the core belief is true, you might not notice evidence that it isn't true.

When you feel you have made sufficient progress, you can advance to the final chapter to wrap up your work.

Part V

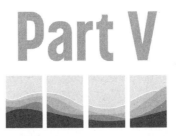

Moving Forward

Congratulations! You have made it to the end of this book! In the final chapters, you'll have the opportunity to reflect on your progress and make plans for what's next for yourself.

16

Finishing Cognitive Processing Therapy

You've worked hard to face your trauma, allowed yourself to experience natural emotions, learned new skills, and evaluated your stuck points. Hopefully you are feeling better and experiencing fewer or less severe symptoms of PTSD. Give yourself a lot of credit for embarking on this difficult work and sticking with it to the end!

Take a moment to reflect on the changes in your life. What changes have you noticed in your work, school, or other productive activities and hobbies?

_____

_____

_____

_____

What changes have you noticed in your relationships with family, friends, coworkers, neighbors, and others?

_____

_____

_____

_____

Have you noticed changes in any other areas of your life, like self-care or health?

_____

_____

_____

_____

Final Impact Statement

Please write at least one page on what you think *now* about why your traumatic event occurred. Also, consider what you think *now* about yourself, others, and the world in the following areas: safety, trust, power/control, esteem, and intimacy.

You can write your responses in the space below.

_____

_____

_____

_____

_____

_____

_____

_____

_____

_____

_____

_____

_____

_____

_____

_____

_____

_____

_____

_____

(continued)

To wrap up your work, you'll be asked to write a Final Impact Statement (see pages 270–271) to reflect on how you think **now**. You can also download and print the Final Impact Statement from *www.guilford.com/resick2-forms*. This exercise will allow you to consider the changes you've made as part of your work in this program. Do this exercise without looking back at your initial Impact Statement, and focus only on what you believe now.

Next, review what you have written in your Final Impact Statement. Then go back and reread what you wrote at the beginning of the book for the first Impact Statement, which you completed in Chapter 4 on pages 47–48.

Reflect on any differences you notice between the two statements. You may be surprised by how much your thinking has changed since you began this process. For example, are there any changes in where you are placing the blame for the trauma? Are your thoughts about safety or trust less extreme? What stands out to you as you compare your statements?

_____

_____

_____

_____

Reflect on the progress you've made as you've worked through this program. Take a look at your Graph for Tracking Your Weekly Scores on page 24 and evaluate any changes in your scores. What are your conclusions? How do you feel now?

_____

_____

_____

_____

Also, look over the items on the Baseline PTSD Checklist on pages 14–15 to notice what specific symptoms have changed. Reflect back on what it was like when you first started this process and how your life has changed since you've improved in those symptoms.

Are there any areas that you think you need to continue working on? For example, are there any stuck points that you may need to do more worksheets on?

_____

_____

_____

_____

Make sure you don't get caught in all-or-none thinking about your progress. Even if there's still more work to do, be sure to celebrate what you've accomplished so far! It took a lot of work to get here! Also, sometimes people who recover from PTSD feel regret that they didn't do this work sooner. If that's something you've thought, consider whether you knew that this kind of help existed, whether it was available to you, and whether you were always in the position you are in now to address your PTSD. It's OK to grieve how much trauma and PTSD have affected your life, but be sure to give yourself credit for the hard work you've put in that's allowed you to move toward recovery and live your life more fully.

Think ahead to goals you might want to accomplish and things that you couldn't do when you were stuck in your PTSD. If you're not feeling as pinned down by the symptoms of PTSD, do you feel like you are now ready to embark on new challenges and opportunities?

Now that you have faced your PTSD, what are your plans for the future?

_____

_____

_____

_____

What goals will you be focusing on next?

_____

_____

_____

_____

Remember that the skills you learned in this book are here for you for the rest of your life. You may be at a point where you can do the worksheets "in your head" without writing, or you may find that it still helps to write them out or to review worksheets you've done previously. If you notice a stuck point that you are really struggling with, try going back and doing an Alternative Thoughts Worksheet on it, even if you've done one on it before or if you normally do them in your head. You may also find that reviewing the chapters on safety, trust, power and control, esteem, and intimacy can help you when you are in challenging situations or times in your life. Remember that the Alternative Thoughts Worksheets can be used for any issues or stressors you have in your life, not just stuck points about your past traumas. The more you practice using the worksheets, the more they become a part of you until you don't need them anymore. The more you practice the alternative thoughts, the more they'll become your new, realistic habit of thinking.

We recommend that you assess how you're doing a month from now. Consider whether you have any remaining stuck points that you are working on or PTSD symptoms that need more attention. You may want to continue working on other traumatic events to see if there are different stuck points you want to address. Some people find it helpful to set aside an hour every week or two to look back over worksheets and complete some new ones on any current issues that are bothering them.

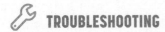 **TROUBLESHOOTING**

What if I'm not feeling better?

Everyone's needs are different. If you had many traumatic events over the course of your life, you may need a bit more time to work on stuck points that are different from those of the index event you started with. If you got off to a slow start (reluctance to do the practice assignments or think about the worst trauma), you may need just a few more weeks to finish up. Just keep practicing and you'll likely soon see improvement in those symptoms. Keep an eye out for all-or-none thinking too. If you feel somewhat but not completely better, that's OK, and it doesn't mean you won't be able to continue to recover.

It's not a failure to need more time and practice. Sometimes people need a few more weeks to do more work on esteem or intimacy because they are such life-changing themes. You may benefit from looking back over the previous chapters with fresh eyes. However, you won't continue this program for an indefinite period of time. You'll usually need just a few more weeks of practice to bring down the remaining PTSD symptoms, and then you can just use the skills when you need them. Going over your responses to the items on the PTSD Checklist may help you determine where you are still stuck. Are you still avoiding certain triggers? What stuck point goes with your avoidance? If you're having nightmares or flashbacks, consider whether there is a part of one of your traumas that has not been processed and what the stuck points and emotions might be.

It's never too late to recover. Different people have different patterns of recovery. Make a commitment to yourself to do everything you can to not avoid anything you've been finding it difficult to talk about, and to make sure you spend time every day on your practice assignments. Celebrate the fact that you have taken steps and made some progress.

If you haven't experienced as much relief from PTSD as you had hoped after a few more weeks, it's important not to give up. You can keep working with these skills and continue to see improvement. You can also seek out a therapist who specializes in CPT. A list of providers in the community is available at *http://cptforptsd.com*. Or, if you are a U.S. veteran, you can ask for a CPT provider at your local Veterans Affairs hospital or clinic. There are also other forms of therapy that can help PTSD. One of them might be a better fit for you. You can learn about them at *www.ptsd.va.gov*. It's important not to give up hope and to keep using all the skills you've been developing.

Will I slide back into my old way of thinking? Am I going to relapse?

The good news is that what you've accomplished in this process is not only changing your thoughts but changing how you think about your thoughts. If you changed your thoughts, you didn't do so just by repeating something overly positive to yourself instead. What you did is you looked at facts and decided what was the most true and fair conclusion. Therefore, you are unlikely to go back to thinking something else that you already decided isn't realistic. However, remember that your old way of thinking may have been a long-ingrained, habitual way of thinking. So, you might sometimes have to remind yourself of the work you did looking at the facts or refer back to your completed worksheets if one of your stuck points pops up. Research has shown us, nonetheless, that people who complete CPT not only change their thinking in the immediate term but also tend to maintain those changes in thinking years later. Likewise, studies have shown that people don't tend to "relapse" with PTSD. Once you have dealt with the trauma, it's unlikely to keep haunting you in the same way. Even if you experience some periods of time where you think about it more or experience some strong feelings when you are reminded of the trauma, you may notice that it feels different now that you have allowed yourself to process the trauma and experience the natural emotions.

What do I do if I have dealt with the worst trauma but still have others?

Often people notice that as they work through their worst trauma, their symptoms and stuck points about other traumas reduce as well. However, if you have stuck points about other traumas, you can continue to use the same skills you applied to the first trauma. Go back to Chapter 7 and the questions there about why the trauma happened. Also continue to use the Alternative Thoughts Worksheets to evaluate your stuck points about your other traumas. You may find that you don't have to spend as much time or do as many worksheets on other traumas, or that it's easier to work on them.

What if I experience a trauma in the future?

There's no way to predict what the future may hold, and we hope that you don't experience another trauma. Still, research has shown us that even if people do have another traumatic event after completing CPT, they are unlikely to experience PTSD again. You've learned new ways to relate to your experiences. You've learned that when something stressful or traumatic happens, it's best not to avoid but to let yourself feel your feelings, talk about it with supportive people, and process your thoughts and emotions. If something stressful or traumatic happens to you in the future, you can use the same set of skills you've already used here to face that experience. Notice any stuck points you have and complete Alternative Thoughts Worksheets on them as needed. You've learned an invaluable skill that you'll have for the rest of your life and can use across many situations.

17

Conclusion

Congratulations on completing this work! This is a major accomplishment that should be celebrated. You faced some very difficult memories, and you devoted a lot of time and effort to your recovery. This took bravery and commitment, and a belief that you could make progress if you did the hard work. Don't forget, or minimize, what it took to do this! Consider completing the certificate on the next page with the date you completed this program as a reminder of your hard work and achievement (or download it from *www.guilford. com/resick2-forms*). As you face the future, you'll take with you all of the important skills that you learned. Keep using them when you need them, and don't forget how much strength and persistence it has taken to face your trauma and take these steps toward recovery from PTSD. We wish you all the best as you continue to move forward.

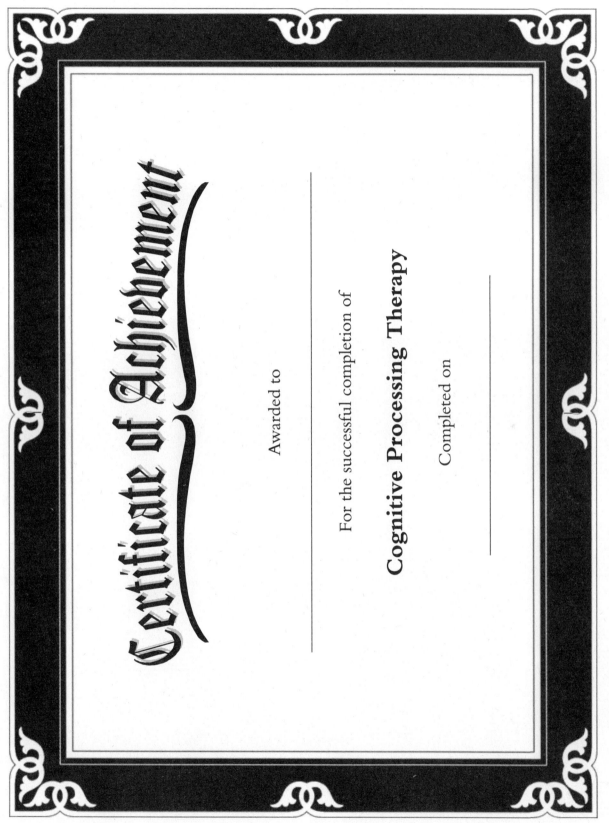

Certificate of Achievement

Awarded to

_____

For the successful completion of

Cognitive Processing Therapy

Completed on

_____

Appendix

On the next page is a handout that you can share with people in your life who you want to support you while you work on CPT.

Following that, you will find the Stuck Point Log for Remaining Stuck Points, which you can use to write down the stuck points you want to continue working on, as well as extra copies of the PTSD Checklist and Alternative Thoughts Worksheet.

The person sharing this with you is working on a self-guided course of cognitive processing therapy (CPT). CPT is an effective treatment for posttraumatic stress disorder (PTSD). Dozens of studies have shown that CPT can help people with their recovery from PTSD. It works by helping people recognize how trauma has changed their view about themselves, others, and the world. CPT teaches people to recognize the negative thoughts that have resulted from trauma. We call them "stuck points" because they get in the way of recovery from PTSD and keep people stuck. Stuck points don't reflect the full context or reality, and CPT works by teaching people how to think through their stuck points and consider new, more true and balanced perspectives. CPT also helps people break the cycle of avoidance that can maintain PTSD. By allowing themselves to do this work rather than avoiding memories, they can process the trauma and begin to recover.

There are four phases of CPT: (1) education about PTSD and CPT; (2) processing the trauma; (3) learning to examine thoughts about the trauma; and (4) examining stuck points related to safety, trust, power and control, esteem, and intimacy.

You can help your loved one by learning more about PTSD. The National Center for PTSD has some helpful resources: *www.ptsd.va.gov/family/how_help_cpt.asp.* You can also ask them if they would like you to support them by reminding them about some of the practice and exercises they'll be doing. If they do, encourage them, but remember that it's not your job to get them to do the work. At times as people do CPT or other forms of trauma treatment, they may experience emotions they've been avoiding, like sadness. This is because they are processing the trauma instead of avoiding. These feelings will decrease over time and become less intense. You can also let them know that you're there to talk and support them, but respect their wishes if they don't want to share much information with you.

It doesn't help to suggest that they stop doing the work if they are feeling bad, because this encourages them to continue avoiding. Instead, let them know that you see how hard they are working and that if they keep it up and get through the tough parts, they can start to see change, or just let them know you're there and that you support them. This book contains other resources and information about what to do if they aren't feeling better or if they're experiencing suicidal thoughts, so if you have concerns about how they're doing, suggest they look over that section.

Your support means a lot to your loved ones when they're working through traumatic events. Thank you for being there and supporting them as they take these steps in their recovery.

Stuck Point Log for Remaining Stuck Points

Stuck point   Alternative thought

_____

_____

_____

_____

_____

_____

_____

_____

_____

_____

_____

_____

_____

_____

_____

_____

_____

_____

_____

_____

_____

_____

_____

(PTSD Checklist)

Complete the PTSD Checklist to track your symptoms. Be sure to complete this measure on the same index event each time. When the instructions and questions refer to a "stressful experience," remember that that is your index event.

Write in here the trauma that you are working on: _____

Complete this PTSD Checklist with reference to that event.

Instructions: Below is a list of problems that people sometimes have in response to a very stressful experience. Please read each problem carefully, and then circle one of the numbers to the right to indicate how much you have been bothered by that problem *in the past week*.

In the past week, how much were you bothered by:	Not at all	A little bit	Mod-erately	Quite a bit	Extremely
1. Repeated, disturbing, and unwanted memories of the stressful experience?	0	1	2	3	4
2. Repeated, disturbing dreams of the stressful experience?	0	1	2	3	4
3. Suddenly feeling or acting as if the stressful experience were actually happening again (*as if you were actually back there reliving it*)?	0	1	2	3	4
4. Feeling very upset when something reminded you of the stressful experience?	0	1	2	3	4
5. Having strong physical reactions when something reminded you of the stressful experience (*for example, heart pounding, trouble breathing, sweating*)?	0	1	2	3	4
6. Avoiding memories, thoughts, or feelings related to the stressful experience?	0	1	2	3	4
7. Avoiding external reminders of the stressful experience (*for example, people, places, conversations, activities, objects, or situations*)?	0	1	2	3	4
8. Trouble remembering important parts of the stressful experience (not due to head injury or substances)?	0	1	2	3	4
9. Having strong negative beliefs about yourself, other people, or the world (*for example, having thoughts such as I am bad, There is something seriously wrong with me, No one can be trusted, or The world is completely dangerous*)?	0	1	2	3	4
10. Blaming yourself or someone else (who didn't intend the outcome) for the stressful experience or what happened after it?	0	1	2	3	4
11. Having strong negative feelings, such as fear, horror, anger, guilt, or shame?	0	1	2	3	4
12. Loss of interest in activities that you used to enjoy?	0	1	2	3	4
13. Feeling distant or cut off from other people?	0	1	2	3	4
14. Trouble experiencing positive feelings (*for example, being unable to feel happiness or have loving feelings for people close to you*)?	0	1	2	3	4
15. Irritable behavior, angry outbursts, or acting aggressively?	0	1	2	3	4
16. Taking too many risks or doing things that could cause you harm?	0	1	2	3	4
17. Being "super alert" or watchful or on guard?	0	1	2	3	4
18. Feeling jumpy or easily startled?	0	1	2	3	4
19. Having difficulty concentrating?	0	1	2	3	4
20. Trouble falling or staying asleep?	0	1	2	3	4

Add up the total and write it here: _____

From *PTSD Checklist for DSM-5 (PCL-5)* by Weathers, Litz, Keane, Palmieri, Marx, and Schnurr (2013). Available from the National Center for PTSD at *www.ptsd.va.gov*; in the public domain. Reprinted in *Getting Unstuck from PTSD* (Guilford Press, 2023). Purchasers of this book can photocopy and/or download additional copies of this worksheet at *www.guilford.com/resick2-forms* for personal use or use with clients; see copyright page for details.

Alternative Thoughts Worksheet

A. Situation	B. Stuck point	C. Emotion(s)	D. Exploring thoughts	E. Thinking patterns	F. Alternative thought(s)
Describe the event leading to the stuck point or unpleasant emotion(s).	Write your stuck point related to the situation in Section A. Rate your belief in this stuck point from 0 to 100%. (How strongly do you believe this thought?)	Specify your emotion(s) (sad, angry, etc.) and rate how strongly you feel each emotion from 0 to 100%.	Use the **exploring questions** to examine your automatic thought from Section B. Consider whether the thought is balanced and factual or extreme. Evidence against? What information is not included? All or none? Extreme? Focused on just one piece of the event? Questionable source of information? Confusing possible with definite? Based on feelings or facts?	Use the **thinking patterns** to decide whether this is one of the patterns and explain why. Jumping to conclusions: Ignoring important parts: Oversimplifying/overgeneralizing: Mind reading: Emotional reasoning:	What else can you say instead of the thought in Section B? How else can you interpret the event instead of this thought? Rate your belief in the alternative thought(s) from 0 to 100%. **G. Re-rate old stuck point** Re-rate how much you now believe the stuck point in Section B from 0 to 100%. **H. Emotion(s)** Now what do you feel? Rate from 0 to 100%.

Alternative Thoughts Worksheet

A. Situation	B. Stuck point	C. Emotion(s)	D. Exploring thoughts	E. Thinking patterns	F. Alternative thought(s)
Describe the event leading to the stuck point or unpleasant emotion(s).	Write your stuck point related to the situation in Section A. Rate your belief in this stuck point from 0 to 100%. (How strongly do you believe this thought?)	Specify your emotion(s) (sad, angry, etc.) and rate how strongly you feel each emotion from 0 to 100%.	Use the **exploring questions** to examine your automatic thought from Section B. Consider whether the thought is balanced and factual or extreme.	Use the **thinking patterns** to decide whether this is one of the patterns and explain why.	What else can you say instead of the thought in Section B? How else can you interpret the event instead of this thought? Rate your belief in the alternative thought(s) from 0 to 100%.
			Evidence against?	Jumping to conclusions:	
			What information is not included?	Ignoring important parts:	
			All or none? Extreme?		
			Focused on just one piece of the event?	Oversimplifying/overgeneralizing:	
			Questionable source of information?	Mind reading:	
			Confusing possible with definite?		
			Based on feelings or facts?	Emotional reasoning:	**G. Re-rate old stuck point** Re-rate how much you now believe the stuck point in Section B from 0 to 100%.
					H. Emotion(s) Now what do you feel? Rate from 0 to 100%.

From *Getting Unstuck from PTSD* by Patricia A. Resick, Shannon Wiltsey Stirman, and Stefanie T. LoSavio. Copyright © 2023 The Guilford Press. Purchasers of this book can photocopy and/or download additional copies of this worksheet at www.guilford.com/resick2-forms for personal use or use with clients; see copyright page for details.

Alternative Thoughts Worksheet

A. Situation	B. Stuck point		D. Exploring thoughts	E. Thinking patterns	F. Alternative thought(s)
Describe the event leading to the stuck point or unpleasant emotion(s).	Write your stuck point related to the situation in Section A. Rate your belief in this stuck point from 0 to 100%. (How strongly do you believe this thought?)		Use the **exploring questions** to examine your automatic thought from Section B. Consider whether the thought is balanced and factual or extreme.	Use the **thinking patterns** to decide whether this is one of the patterns and explain why.	What else can you say instead of the thought in Section B? How else can you interpret the event instead of this thought? Rate your belief in the alternative thought(s) from 0 to 100%.
			Evidence against?	Jumping to conclusions:	
			What information is not included?	Ignoring important parts:	
			All or none? Extreme?		
			Focused on just one piece of the event?	Oversimplifying/overgeneralizing:	
	C. Emotion(s) Specify your emotion(s) (sad, angry, etc.) and rate how strongly you feel each emotion from 0 to 100%.		Questionable source of information?	Mind reading:	**G. Re-rate old stuck point** Re-rate how much you now believe the stuck point in Section B from 0 to 100%.
			Confusing possible with definite?		
			Based on feelings or facts?	Emotional reasoning:	**H. Emotion(s)** Now what do you feel? Rate from 0 to 100%.

Resources

In this section you'll find some additional information and resources that may be helpful. We've included a list of some common stuck points for people with specific types of trauma histories, as well as some questions that may be helpful to ask yourself about specific stuck points you may have.

~~~~~~~~~~~~~~~~~ Additional Tools ~~~~~~~~~~~~~~~~~

Common Stuck Points for Specific Trauma Types

Childhood Sexual Abuse

- I must have done something that made them think I wanted it.
- They picked me for a reason (something about me specifically).
- I should have told someone that the abuse was going on.
- I should have told someone sooner that the abuse was going on.
- I wasn't worth protecting.
- I shouldn't have liked the attention.
- I should have said "No."
- I should have fought back.
- I should have run away.
- It happened because I hugged that person/sat on their lap.
- I shouldn't have done what they told me to do.
- I must have wanted it/liked it.

Childhood Physical Abuse

- It happened because I was bad.
- I did something to deserve the abuse.
- It happened because I was unlovable.
- I wasn't worth taking care of/protecting.
- I should have told someone.
- I should have run away.
- I should have fought back.
- Maybe it wasn't really abuse.

Adult Sexual Assault

- I should have fought harder.
- I should have said "No."
- I let it happen.
- I shouldn't have froze.
- I shouldn't have been in that situation (drinking, out alone, etc.).

- I should have known that person would assault me.
- It happened because I flirted.

- It happened because of the way I looked/dressed.
- Maybe it wasn't really a rape.
- They must have thought I wanted it.

Adult Physical Assault/Abuse

- I should have seen the red flags that this person was an abuser.
- I should have left them the first time it happened.
- It happened because of something I did wrong.

- I shouldn't have provoked them.
- If I had been a better partner, they wouldn't have abused me.
- I should have been more careful.
- It happened because of my bad judgment.

Traumatic Loss (Such as War, Suicide, Drug Overdose, Murder)

- I should have known that this was going to happen.
- I should have done more to help.
- I should have been there.
- If I had done something different, they would still be here.
- I wasn't worth them living for/getting clean for.

- I will never get over losing that person.
- I can't go on without them.
- I should have gotten them out of that situation while there was still time.
- I should have protected my loved ones/the children I saw/others.

Combat

- It should have been me who got hurt/killed instead of them.
- I shouldn't have felt exhilarated while [the traumatic event] was happening.
- That's not how combat/service is supposed to be (hidden explosives, enemies firing from a distance, children or women as combatants or decoys, friendly fire, training accidents, etc.).
- We should have been able to do more.

- The enemy attack was our commanding officer's fault.
- I shouldn't have enlisted/accepted that post.
- I shouldn't have fired on those people.
- If I had been a better leader, it wouldn't have happened.
- I should have been there the day it happened.
- I shouldn't have felt as terrified as I felt.
- I shouldn't have frozen/I should have reacted more quickly.

Trauma Secondary to Work as a First Responder (as in Medic, Firefighter, or Police Officer)

- I should have been able to save that person.
- I failed them.
- I should have been faster.

- It's my fault that the person died.
- If I were more competent, I would have saved them.

Trauma Associated with Being a Medical Professional

- I made the wrong call.
- It happened because I didn't react quickly enough.
- I should have been able to save them.
- I should have responded faster.
- It's all the fault of [the hospital system/a coworker].
- I should have been kinder to that patient.
- I should have spoken up when I saw something going wrong.

Trauma Associated with Being a Refugee

- I should have left sooner.
- I shouldn't have left at all.
- I should have brought more family members with me.
- I should have persuaded my loved ones to come with me.
- I should have been able to protect my loved ones.
- I will never be able to move on.
- Things like this are not supposed to happen.
- I shouldn't recover while others are still suffering.

Questions to Consider for Common Stuck Points

"I should have seen the red flags that this person was an abuser."

- What were your original impressions of the person?
- How did they originally treat you?
- What signs are you thinking you should have seen? Were there really any? Did you notice signs at the time? What did you think about those facts then?
- Are there any reasons that you might not have trusted your instincts, such as previous violations that caused you to doubt yourself or your feelings?

"I should have left the first time it happened."

- What were the reasons you didn't leave?
- At the time, what were you thinking or hoping would happen next?
- Did you know then what would happen next, how it would progress, or how long it would go on?

"I should have fought harder."

- What did you do? If you initially fought back, did it work? What happened? Does it make sense that you might have stopped resisting?
- Is it possible that if you fought harder, the outcome would have been the same, such as that it was not possible to overcome the other person?
- Is it possible that if you fought harder, you could have been hurt worse or killed?

"I should have said 'No.'"

- What did you say?
- Did you say "Yes"?
- What did your body language say?
- If someone were to react the way you did, would you keep going?

"I let the event happen."

- Did you *want* the event to happen?
- Did you *intend* for it to happen?
- *Let* implies that you had control. How much control did you actually have?

"I should have told someone."

- What were the reasons you did not tell someone?
- How were you feeling at the time?
- How old were you? Is it reasonable that someone your age in your situation would not tell (for example, because of feelings of fear, or not knowing who to tell or what to say?)?
- What were you hoping would happen next?
- Is it possible that even if you told, it might have continued anyway?

"It happened because I was bad."

- What did you do that was "bad"? Does the punishment seem fair?
- Do other people do the same things you did without experiencing the trauma you experienced?
- Would you punish someone the way you were for the same thing you did? Would you make the punishment that extreme?
- Does the response say more about you or the perpetrator?
- Where did you get the idea that you were bad? Consider the source. Is this a "just-world" belief?

"It happened because I was unlovable."

- What was "unlovable" about you? Would you consider other people with those traits or behaviors to be completely unlovable? Would you think they deserved to experience what you experienced?
- Is anyone truly unlovable?
- Does the abuse say more about you or the perpetrator?
- Is that the conclusion you came to in childhood and never questioned it?

"I shouldn't have been in that situation."

- What were the reasons that you were you in that situation? What were your intentions when you went into the situation?
- Did you know then what was going to happen?
- Had you been in that situation before with a different outcome? Does being in that situation always cause that outcome?
- When you focus on being in the situation, are you leaving out any other factors that needed to be in place for the trauma to occur (such as someone intending to hurt you)?

"I should have protected other people."

- Was it really possible to protect other people in the moment?
- What was going on that prevented you from protecting them?
- Did you make a decision not to protect others in the moment or did it happen too quickly? If you made a decision, what were the reasons?

~~~~~~~~~~ Additional Places to Get Information or Help ~~~~~~~~~~

Guilford website with downloadable CPT forms: *www.guilford.com/resick2-forms*
CPT for PTSD website (Whiteboard video library, list of therapists trained in CPT, research
    articles): *https://cptforptsd.com*
National Center for PTSD: *www.ptsd.va.gov*
National Domestic Violence Hotline: *www.thehotline.org*
PTSD Coach mobile app: *www.ptsd.va.gov/appvid/mobile/ptsdcoach_app.asp*

Suicide Prevention Resources

United States

National Suicide Prevention Lifeline: 988; *www.988lifeline.org*

United Kingdom

Emergency services (police, fire, ambulance): 999
Free national nongovernmental helpline available 24/7: *www.samaritans.org*

Australia

Emergency services: 000
National suicide/crisis service is called Lifeline: *www.lifeline.org.au* and people can call it (13 11 14)
    or chat or text them (see the website for those links).

Canada

Emergency services: 911
National Suicide Hotline: 800-273-8255
Talk Suicide Canada: *www.crisisservicescanada.ca*

Index

About the Authors

Patricia A. Resick, PhD, ABPP, is Professor Emeritus of Psychiatry and Behavioral Sciences at Duke University School of Medicine. Dr. Resick first developed CPT in 1988 and has trained thousands of therapists, including the coauthors of this book, to use CPT with their clients. Dr. Resick is a recipient of Lifetime Achievement Awards from the International Society for Traumatic Stress Studies, the Association for Behavioral and Cognitive Therapies, and the Trauma Psychology Division of the American Psychological Association, among other honors.

Shannon Wiltsey Stirman, PhD, is Professor of Psychiatry and Behavioral Sciences at Stanford University. She has been working with people with PTSD and conducting research on PTSD since the early 2000s. Dr. Wiltsey Stirman provides training and consultation in CPT and cognitive-behavioral therapy.

Stefanie T. LoSavio, PhD, ABPP, is Assistant Professor of Psychiatry and Behavioral Sciences at the University of Texas Health Science Center at San Antonio and Director of Research and Innovation at the STRONG STAR Training Initiative. Dr. LoSavio specializes in evidence-based treatments for PTSD and is a CPT researcher, trainer, and consultant.